Healthcare: A Better Way

The New Era of Opportunity

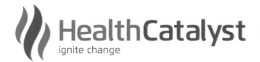

ACKNOWLEDGMENTS

Sir Isaac Newton is known to have said, "If I have seen further it is by standing on the shoulders of giants." This certainly captures the circumstances of this book. The intent of the book is to provide the reader a concise overview of the challenges facing healthcare, the emerging solutions to those challenges and a glimpse of an exciting new future for our noble profession. As such, the book represents very little original thought on my part. Rather, it is a compilation of the works of many visionary leaders that I have had the good fortune of encountering throughout my professional career. I am deeply indebted to each of these great leaders for sharing their wisdom, insights and experience.

My good friend Brent James, MD, is a deeply inspirational leader who has patiently and steadfastly worked for three decades to improve healthcare and inspire healthcare leaders both nationally and internationally. He has had an immense impact on me and on countless others. David Burton, MD, recognized the importance of quality improvement early in his career, and through his visionary leadership as both a clinician and an operational leader he demonstrated that quality improvement could be successfully integrated into the complex process of care delivery. I do not know any two clinicians who have demonstrated this more effectively in a real-world care delivery environment than David and Brent. Robert Wachter, MD, has had a greater impact on increasing awareness of the issues related to patient safety and done more to advance the cause of patient safety than any physician leader I know. Bob's book on patient safety, "Understanding Patient Safety" (Second Edition), is the quintessential resource on this important topic. Along with Brent James, my dear friend, Molly Coye, MD, co-authored the seminal Institute of Medicine (IOM) reports To Err Is Human and Crossing the Quality Chasm. Molly has contributed greatly to advancing awareness of quality in healthcare and to our understanding of the role of emerging technologies in the future of care delivery. Steve Barlow, Tom Burton and Dale Sanders are phenomenally creative leaders in information technology (IT) and healthcare analytics, and they have incredibly deep experience in architecting and deploying successful technology and analytics solutions. Holly Rimmasch, RN, has two decades of experience in improving clinical care, including implementation of clinical and operational best practices. Cherbon VanEtten is knowledgeable in IT, analytics, clinical operations and education. She was a valuable member of the editing team. Dan Burton, the CEO of Health Catalyst, is an imaginative, kind, intelligent and supportive leader who has skillfully guided Health Catalyst to ever-increasing success. Dan also had the wisdom and courage to support this project. Paul Horstmeier has launched and grown three different businesses and won numerous industry awards for quality and innovation. It is healthcare's good fortune that Dan and Paul are now applying their deep experience to transforming healthcare. Leslie Falk, RN, provided her experience in healthcare, business, writing and

editing. Leslie has been a joy to work with on this project. Sister Monica Heeran, CSJP, is one of the most supportive and thoughtful leaders I have ever known. Without her vision and willingness to take a risk with a young physician leader, my career would never have been the same. John Hayward has been a longtime mentor and friend. He has more passion for improving healthcare than any non-clinician that I have ever known. I am indebted to Elaine Dunda and Donn McMillan. Working alongside Elaine and Donn, I was able to gain deep, pragmatic experience in successfully implementing quality and safety into a complex integrated care delivery environment.
Last, but certainly far from least, I would like to recognize the thousands of clinical and operational leaders across the country who are daring greatly and working tirelessly to improve care for patients and communities. They are an inspiration to all of us.

These are the shoulders on which I stand and on which this book is built.

John L. Haughom, MD

CONTENTS

PART TWO:
LAYING THE FOUNDATION FOR IMPROVEMENT AND SUSTAINABLE CHANGE

CHAPTER FIVE: THE DEPLOYMENT SYSTEM: STANDARD ORGANIZATIONAL WORK 95

CHAPTER SIX: THE CONTENT SYSTEM: STANDARD KNOWLEDGE WORK 119

PART THREE:
LOOKING INTO THE FUTURE

INTRODUCTION

Daring greatly

To have lived through a revolution, to have seen a new birth of science, a new dispensation of health, reorganized medical schools, remodeled hospitals, a new outlook for humanity, is an opportunity not given to every generation.

Sir William Osler (1849–1919)

The great Sir William Osler wrote these words in April 1913, near the end of his career and six years before he died. He lived and practiced during a time of great change in healthcare. Over the roughly three decades between 1880 and 1915, Sir William and a few dozen other visionary clinicians laid the foundation for modern clinical care. The physical layout and operational structure of the modern hospital was initially defined. The basic four-year medical school curriculum (two years of basic science and two years of on the ward clinical experience) was established. Postgraduate educational requirements were articulated. Strict licensure requirements for physicians were put into place. The first textbooks of medicine and surgery were written. Scientific research was made the foundation for clinical practice. Foundations for modern nursing practices were created. New hygiene practices to prevent infection were implemented.

Over the past century, we have clearly enhanced and improved these practices and added new advances. Yet, it remains true that we owe a great debt to these visionary clinicians. We are still living their legacy. There was a need for change. These visionary leaders rose to the challenge and charted a new course for healthcare that has lasted more than a century and remains the basis for the way care is provided around the world.

Our turn to create a new vision

This is a difficult and challenging time in healthcare. Once again, we are facing a profound need for change. Anyone involved in leadership and the practice of care knows this is the case. We face an unprecedented level of complexity that is overwhelming our systems and the people trying to practice within them. Far too many outcomes are inadequate. While "first do no harm" is our mantra, we know that the level of harm patients experience when seeking our services is not acceptable. According to the Institute of Medicine (IOM), an estimated 44,000 to 98,000 deaths per year result from avoidable harm. Costs are out of control and waste is widespread. Far too many people lack access to basic health services. The list goes on.

The healthcare world is changing, and for good reason. Now it is our turn to create a new vision and chart a new course for clinical care and for health. Certainly, anyone involved in healthcare leadership, and arguably everyone involved in healthcare, should participate. Clinicians have a professional responsibility to be involved. This is the foundation of why we exist. Physicians, nurses and other care providers need to change the system. We need to create a system of care delivery that allows those working in it — in collaboration with patients — to achieve its potential on behalf of the patients and communities we serve. While many will be involved in this transformative endeavor, it will not be any different than 100 years ago. Pioneering clinical leaders can — and must — lead the way. They have the knowledge of clinical care and the focus on patients that is necessary to successfully lead change. We need to stand on the shoulders of giants to glimpse — and create — a new and better future for healthcare. Working to improve patient care is a noble cause of the first order.

> The healthcare world is changing, and for good reason. Now it is our turn to create a new vision and chart a new course for clinical care and for health.

One can make an effective argument that we have adequate resources. However, those resources are definitely not being efficiently used to meet the care requirements of those in need in our society. Organizations need to improve access to and the consistency, quality, safety and cost of care, in addition to eliminating unnecessary waste. Accomplishing this requires a deep understanding of clinical and operational processes in addition to an ability to design, adopt, implement and manage new, more efficient care delivery processes and care delivery models. While this will require a true multidisciplinary, highly collaborative approach, real success will mandate the passionate engagement of clinical leaders and front-line clinicians. Without capturing the hearts and minds of clinicians, it will be very difficult for any organization to successfully negotiate the tumultuous changes over the next few years. Thus, while this educational resource is designed to inform and engage many stakeholders, it is particularly aimed at informing and engaging physicians, nurses and other healthcare providers.

Knowledge source for those who dare greatly

This book represents the compilation of the works of many. It is designed to be a knowledge source for clinical and operational leaders, as well as front-line caregivers, who are involved in improving processes, reducing harm, designing and implementing new care delivery models, and generally undertaking the difficult task of leading meaningful change on behalf of the patients we serve. It is designed to be a living document. This generation's healthcare leaders need to frame the need for change in language and with logic that appeals to the values of stakeholders. They also need to articulate a compelling new vision for care, explain how that vision will be achieved, and help individual stakeholders understand their role in achieving and sustaining this new vision. It is hoped this book will be a resource for leaders engaged in this critically important change endeavor. While this book may eventually appear in some paper-based form, it is purposely starting out as a digital document and will remain primarily so. This will allow frequent updates and adaptations as events rapidly unfold and progress is made.

Thanks to some pioneering individuals and organizations, we can now see enough of the future of healthcare to have a sense of what it will be. And it is exciting. Empowering. Better for patients and communities. The new ideas, vision, tools and methods capable of supporting meaningful change are falling into place. As progress is made, the digital format of this book will allow it to evolve as rapidly and often as necessary. In that sense, this book will never be done, nor should it be. Like all of healthcare, this is a knowledge tool that should be, and will be, a continuous improvement experience.

No doubt, this is a time of adversity in healthcare. As hard as it is, one can view adversity as a privilege and an opportunity. During times of great change and adversity, we cannot control circumstances, but we can change how we view them. We need to lean into the adversity. Many involved in the healthcare profession need to see a glimpse of the future, understand their role in it and be sustained by a sense of hope. It is our responsibility — and privilege — to offer this to them.

Three years before Sir William wrote the quote at the beginning of this introduction, Theodore Roosevelt delivered the following words in a speech:

> *It is not the critic who counts; not the man who points out how the strong man stumbles, or where the doer of deeds could have done them better. The credit belongs to the man who is actually in the arena, whose face is marred by dust and sweat and blood; who strives valiantly; who errs, who comes short again and again, because there is no effort without error and shortcoming; but who does actually strive to do the deeds; who knows great enthusiasms, the great devotions; who spends himself in a worthy cause; who at the best knows in the end the triumph of high achievement, and who at the worst, if he fails, at least fails while daring greatly, so that his place shall never be with those cold and timid souls who neither know victory nor defeat.*

> *Theodore Roosevelt, 1910*

This quote is certainly pertinent to the situation we currently face in healthcare. We are experiencing one of those "opportunities not often given" described by Sir William. Change is hard, and those of us involved in it feel how hard it is. If Sir William — and other early pioneers — were alive today,

I am confident they would look around and say, "Ah yes … — yes. This is where we need to be." This is where we need to be as well. We need to stay in the arena and "dare greatly."

So, welcome to the arena. I am glad to be here with you. I hope the information in this dynamic book helps you see and prepare for an exciting new future.

I invite you to join me in making this book the best support tool it can be.

John L. Haughom, MD
February 2014

PART ONE: FORCES DRIVING TRANSFORMATION

Introduction

Over the past decade, much has been written about the problems with healthcare in the United States. While the need to improve quality and decrease costs is real, it is important to not forget what is good about our healthcare system. The purpose of part 1 is to provide an overview of the historical, cultural, financial and social forces that have defined and shaped the existing healthcare system and the dynamics that are irreversibly driving the need for change. This will set the stage for part 2, which reviews emerging concepts and methods that will allow healthcare organizations to adapt to a rapidly changing future.

1 FORCES DEFINING AND SHAPING THE CURRENT STATE OF U.S. HEALTHCARE

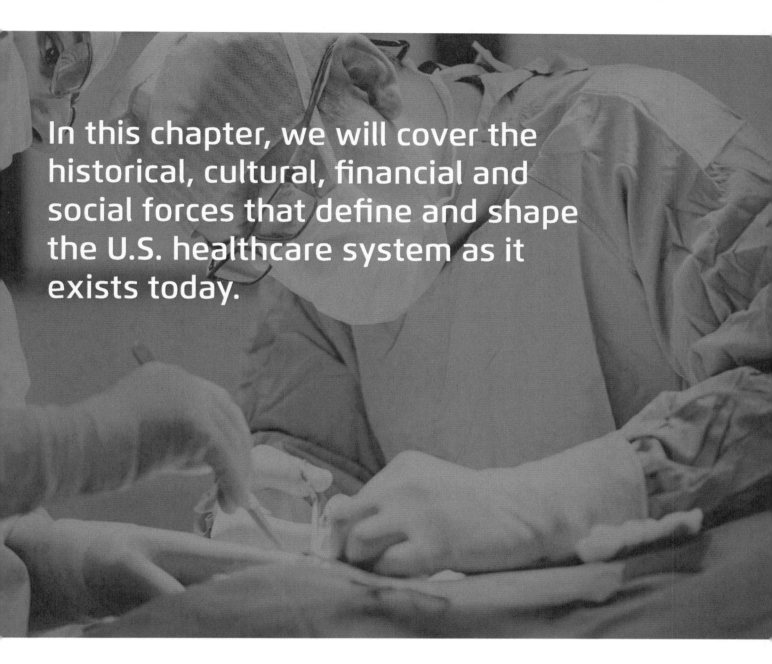

In this chapter, we will cover the historical, cultural, financial and social forces that define and shape the U.S. healthcare system as it exists today.

What's good about U.S. healthcare: 100 years of progress

We hear a lot lately about the problems with healthcare in the United States. While the need to improve quality and decrease costs is real, let's not forget to celebrate what is good about our healthcare system. It is worthwhile to briefly review the past 100 years of history to emphasize one point: our healthcare is the best the world has ever seen!

Consider these simple examples:

- From 1900 to 2010, average life expectancy at birth increased from only 49 years to almost 80 years.[1]

- Since 1960, age-adjusted mortality from heart disease (the #1 cause of death) has decreased by 56 percent.[2]

- Since 1950, age-adjusted mortality from stroke has decreased by 70 percent.[3]

Why so much progress over the last 100 years? Let's explore a few of the historical trends.

The emergence of modern medicine

For much of history, if you were ill or injured and saw a physician, your chances of survival actually went down. Hospitals were the places where people went to die. Actually, hospitals were the places where the poor went to die. If you had any resources at all, you invited a physician into your home … and you died at home.

Just prior to 1900, this all changed profoundly as a result of the vision and hard work of a handful of visionary clinical leaders (William Osler, William Halsted, Howard Kelly, Florence Nightingale, William Welch, Harvey Cushing, etc.). It is possible to credit the change to a handful of impactful advances in the medical profession:

- New, high standards of clinical education

- Strict requirements for professional licensing

- Clinical practice founded on scientific research

- New internal organization for hospitals

- Creation of new, more modern nurse practices

- Implementation of more modern hygiene techniques

- New public health policies and treatments

Since that time, we in the medical profession routinely achieve miracles.

A century of strides in public health and patient care

It is illuminating to look at the change in life expectancy in the U.S. since 1900. Figure 1 shows that a child born in 1900 had a life expectancy just shy of 50 years. For a child born 110 years later, the life expectancy is 78 years — an increase of over 28 years! This is an amazing accomplishment and, frankly, something unseen in the prior 6,000 years of recorded human history (where life expectancy remained relatively flat).[1]

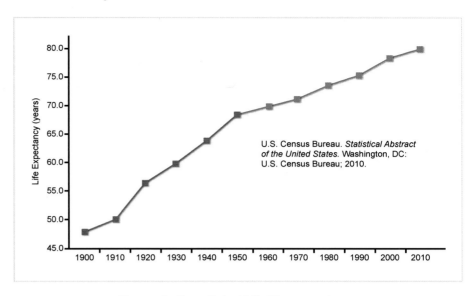

Figure 1: Growth in U.S. life expectancy

Much of this increase can be attributed to improvements in public health. That's why the first half of the 20th century could be called the Public Health Era. Advances in public health led to a gain of about 3.5 years in life expectancy with each passing decade. The increase was largely due to avoiding epidemics of infectious disease such as cholera, typhus and smallpox.

Then, sometime between 1950 and 1960, two things happened:

1. We largely exhausted (though not completely) public health as a major source of increase in life expectancy.

2. For the first time, we began to document gains in life expectancy in the population as a whole from treatment provided in hospitals and clinics. You'll notice that the curve on the graph flattens out a bit at this point — a gain of about 1.3 years of life expectancy per decade. Though less than the public health increase, against the sweep of human history, the gain driven by clinical care is still phenomenal.

We stand on the foundation of 100 years of science that has massively improved our understanding of the human organism in health and disease and given us thousands of ways to improve the well-being and life expectancy of patients.

Only in the last 60 years have we been able to show that clinical care can make a difference. This is in the lifetime of many people involved in healthcare today. We can do more than just predict whether a patient will live or die. **We can actually change the outcome.** We are the first generation of clinicians that can make that claim. That's something that I'm proud and excited to be a part of.

Does history matter?

All of this history is important because it changes how we think about the present and future. No doubt, we face many challenges. As healthcare increasingly contributes to the national debate, let's debate in the context of the phenomenal progress we've made and the progress we're capable of making. And let's remember that at least 95 percent of our peer clinicians get up every day seeking to be the best they can be for the patients they serve. They have a deep-seated professional expertise and a passion for quality that can be tapped as we seek to address the challenges and transform the system.

The primary determinants of health: The Great Equation is wrong

It is not hard to make the case that American healthcare is the best the world has ever seen. However, it is also easy to effectively argue that there is vast room for improvement. Paradoxically, the profession is falling significantly short of its theoretical potential. This does not negate the obvious advances made over the past century, but it is important to understand this reality because it is the source of much of the current criticism.

The healthcare Great Equation

In 1977, Aaron Wildavsky, an American political scientist known for his work on public policy, published a book entitled "Doing Better and Feeling Worse: The Political Pathology of Health Policy."[4] In the book, Wildavsky argued that the traditional belief that "medical care equals health," the so called "Great Equation," simply wasn't true. Most of the bad things that happen to people are at present beyond the reach of medicine. More available medical care does not equal better health.

Determinants of how well we live

One of the most-cited statistics in public health is the imbalance of social investments in medical care compared with prevention activities. Approximately 95 percent of the trillions of dollars we spend as a nation on health goes to direct medical care services, while just 5 percent is allocated to population-wide approaches to health improvement.[5] However, some 40 percent of deaths are caused by behavior patterns that could be modified by preventive interventions as shown in Figure 2. Genetics, social circumstances and environmental exposure also contribute substantially to preventable illness. It appears, in fact, that a much smaller proportion of preventable mortality in the United States, perhaps 10–15 percent, could be avoided by better availability or quality of medical care. Thus, one could question a funding scheme that places so much emphasis on medical care rather than prevention.

The fact that medical care historically has had limited impact on the health of populations has been known for many years. The data clearly indicates we could achieve a much greater impact on total health by going after behaviors than by delivering care.

To put this in perspective, a study published in the British Medical Journal tracked approximately 35,000 people over about 20 years.[6] The study looked at 4 behaviors related to health (tobacco use, appropriate alcohol use, diet and exercise) and demonstrated that people who did well on all 4 compared to people who did poorly on all four accounted for a 14-year difference in life expectancy. Compare this to all of healthcare delivery accounting for approximately 3.5 to 7 years of additional life expectancy.

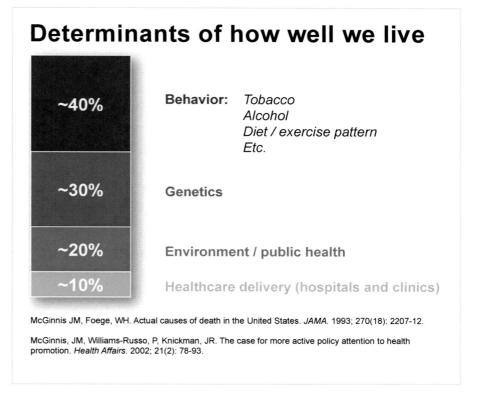

Determinants of how well we live

~40%   **Behavior:**   *Tobacco*
                        Alcohol
                        Diet / exercise pattern
                        Etc.

~30%   **Genetics**

~20%   **Environment / public health**

~10%   Healthcare delivery (hospitals and clinics)

McGinnis JM, Foege, WH. Actual causes of death in the United States. *JAMA*. 1993; 270(18): 2207-12.

McGinnis, JM, Williams-Russo, P, Knickman, JR. The case for more active policy attention to health promotion. *Health Affairs*. 2002; 21(2): 78-93.

Figure 2: Determinants of how well we live

How this impacts the healthcare policy debate

Doctors have little or no control over 90 percent of factors that determine health, from individual lifestyle (smoking, exercise, worry), to social conditions (income, eating habits, physiological inheritance), to physical environment (air and water quality). Most of the bad things that happen to people are at present beyond the reach of medicine.

Everyone knows that doctors do help patients. We can mend broken bones, cure most infections and successfully operate on diseased organs. Inoculations, infections and organ repairs are good reasons for having doctors, drugs and hospitals available. More of the same, however, is likely counterproductive. Nobody needs unnecessary operations, and excessive use of drugs can create dependencies or adverse reactions resulting in patient harm.

More money for clinical care alone cannot advance health. In the absence of medical knowledge gained through new research, or of administrative and clinical knowledge to advance common practice into best practice, current medicine has gone as far as it can. It will not produce more if more money is applied, and one could argue that we should be advancing anyway, especially with the extensive expenditures that the U.S. already applies to clinical care and the well-defined levels of wasted resources that could be applied to advancing clinical care.

Spending on health is not necessarily bad. Would we rather spend our disposable income on a new car, a more powerful personal computer or a TV instead? The problem is that healthcare spending as a percent of disposable income in the U.S. is growing much faster than disposable income itself is growing (see discussion of healthcare spending below). This growth in healthcare spending is impacting other categories of spending — such as education and other socially beneficial programs. The argument is not that clinical care is bad, only that it is not good for everything. The marginal value of spending an additional dollar — or 1 billion dollars — on medical care is likely to be close to zero in terms of improving health.

A simple look at healthcare inflation demonstrates why this has caused policymakers to increasingly take a very hard look at healthcare costs in the United States. In 1960, per capita health costs in the U.S. were $146. In 2012, the per capita costs exceeded $8,000.[7] While there has been a return on this societal investment, it has not been as great as one would want. In addition, as healthcare costs move beyond 20 percent of gross domestic product (GDP), it is becoming an increasing burden for both the public and private sector. The U.S. spends far more on health as a percent of GDP than other industrialized countries.[8] This is making it hard for the U.S. to compete in an increasingly globalized economy.

The twofold solution

The solution to this national dilemma is twofold:

1. First, we need to slow the rate of growth in spending on healthcare.

2. Second, we have to spend what we devote to healthcare more efficiently. That is, we need to realize greater value from the resources dedicated to clinical care.

Published studies indicate that the rate of waste in healthcare is somewhere between 30 and 50 percent.[9] The causes of waste need to be eliminated. This is where aggressive, data driven process improvement enters the picture. Experience at leading healthcare delivery organizations has clearly shown that clinician-driven performance improvement can improve outcomes, reduce harm, increase patient satisfaction, reduce waste and save large sums of money. Such value-based performance improvement efforts can assure that waste is eliminated and health expenditures are more efficiently used.

In addition, new more efficient, patient-centric, and ambulatory based care delivery models need to be implemented. The National Committee for

Quality Assurance (NCQA) Medical Home is a clear example of this trend. Technology and advanced data management will play a role in enabling these new care models. Several studies have shown that these technology-enabled models of care can reduce the annual costs to manage some high-profile chronic diseases by up to 40 percent. Given that roughly two dozen chronic diseases account for almost 75 percent of U.S. health expenditures, these new models of care offer great potential to address healthcare inflation. They have also been shown to allow clinicians to manage more patients, which will help address a growing clinician shortage, especially of physicians and nurses.

The old equation is wrong. It is time for a new equation. In a world of increasingly constrained resources, individual life cannot be the sole determinate of how we allocate resources.

The Rule of Rescue

In 1986, U.S. bioethicist Albert Jonsen described the so-called "Rule of Rescue."[10] In Jonsen's words:

> *Our moral response to the imminence of death demands that we rescue the doomed. We throw a rope to the drowning, rush into burning buildings to snatch the entrapped, dispatch teams to search for the snowbound. This rescue morality spills over into medical care, where ropes are artificial hearts, our rush is the mobile critical care unit, our teams the transplant services. The imperative to rescue is, undoubtedly, of great moral significance; [...]*

John McKie and Jeff Richardson subsequently defined the Rule of Rescue as "the imperative to rescue identifiable individuals facing avoidable death, without giving much thought to the opportunity cost for doing so."

Note their use of the key phrase "identifiable individuals." The Rule of Rescue describes the moral impulse to save identifiable lives in immediate danger at any expense. Think of the extremes taken to rescue a small child who has fallen down a well, a woman pinned beneath the rubble of an earthquake, or a submarine crew trapped on the ocean floor. In these situations, no effort is deemed too great.

The Rule of Rescue has held particular significance in the United States where the importance of the individual has long been a part of our cultural fabric. In the U.S., we tend to count ourselves as not fully human unless we pull out all the stops. Increasingly, however, healthcare ethicists and policymakers are asking whether this same moral instinct to rescue, regardless of cost, should be applied in the emergency room, the hospital or the community clinic.

Statistics and costs tend not to invoke as much passion among the American public as individual cases of clinical need. For example, it has been estimated that 29,000 children around the world, mostly in poor countries, die every day from readily preventable causes, yet there is no outpouring of media attention, public or private donations or aircraft carriers steaming out to rescue them. We will readily spend hundreds of thousands of dollars on organ transplants and other procedures that may give a few months of limited life to someone, while we don't spend much smaller sums that could prevent many cases of premature illness and death. The estimated cost for prophylactic Factor VIII to treat one patient with hemophilia for one year is $300,000. Costs of this magnitude have been accepted by public and private insurers in the developed world, even though, in principle, these sums could provide greater overall health benefit if allocated to pay for the unmet healthcare needs of many other patients.

Let's look at various forms of "rescue care" by nation, comparing the U.S. to major European countries (France, Germany and the United Kingdom), based on Organization for Economic Cooperation and Development data (OECD, 2009).[11] First, the prevalence of renal dialysis (Figure 3) and kidney transplants for chronic renal failure (Figure 4).

The performance of renal dialysis and renal transplant in major European countries is substantially less than in the U.S. It is not that these countries do not have patients that would benefit from dialysis and transplant.

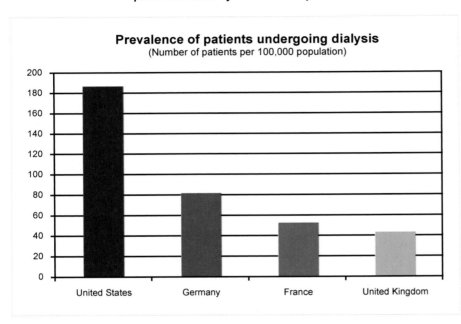

Prevalence of patients undergoing dialysis
(Number of patients per 100,000 population)

Figure 3: Prevalence of patients undergoing dialysis

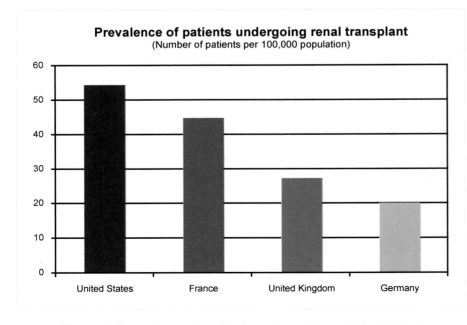

Prevalence of patients undergoing renal transplant
(Number of patients per 100,000 population)

Figure 4: Prevalence of patients undergoing renal transplant

It is a matter of public policy in using renal dialysis and transplant in the treatment of advanced renal failure. The U.S. uses these interventions extensively — European countries much less so.

Now, let's look at the mortality rate from acute myocardial infarction (AMI) in Figure 5, comparing the United States with major European countries.

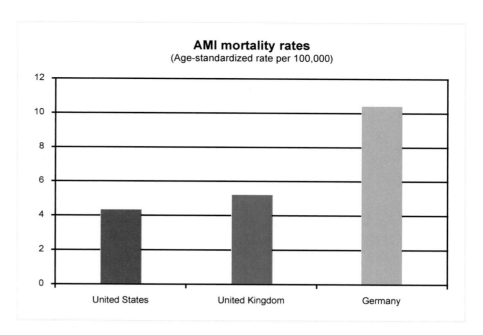

Figure 5: AMI mortality rates 2009

Once again, it is not that the European countries do not have ischemic heart disease. Rather, the point is that AMI is treated much more aggressively with all potential treatment modalities in the United States compared to major European countries.

Finally, let's compare mortality rates from cancer between the United States and major European countries, as shown in Figure 6.

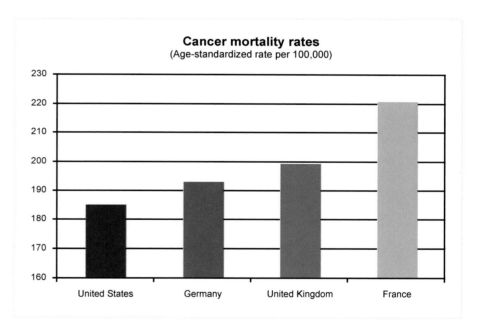

Figure 6: Cancer mortality rates 2009

Cancer is equally prevalent in Europe as it is in the United States, but we tend to treat it much more aggressively here, offering patients every opportunity to be cured, or at least to extend their lives.

Despite spending twice as much as the average Western European country on its healthcare (see discussion on health expenditures below), the United States lags behind on a number of health system performance indicators, including amenable mortality — that is, deaths that could have been avoided with timely and effective healthcare. Examples of such conditions include diabetes and acute infections, as summarized in Figure 7.[12]

The impact on total health

In terms of "total health" as measured by mortality amenable to timely and effective medical care, the U.S. does not do as well. The reason for this discrepancy is that the U.S. does not focus on primary care and prevention. We place a very heavy focus on rescue care. Many countries outperform the U.S. as a result of better public health, a greater focus on behaviors and better primary care. However, the U.S. performs significantly better for those with severe illness or injury (i.e., in terms of rescue care) as a result of better access to technology, less explicit rationing and easy access to subspecialists.

Going forward, as pressure to control healthcare costs grows and the need to manage precious resources more carefully increases, the broad application of the Rule of Rescue will be increasingly untenable. But the cultural and moral instinct to apply it will continue. The desire to help those weakest among us will remain strong, especially when their small numbers allow us to see them as unique individuals. This will likely be a very difficult cultural norm for American society to manage as healthcare transformation unfolds.

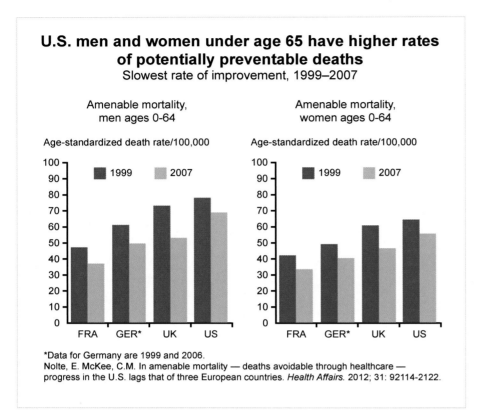

U.S. men and women under age 65 have higher rates of potentially preventable deaths
Slowest rate of improvement, 1999–2007

Amenable mortality, men ages 0-64

Amenable mortality, women ages 0-64

Age-standardized death rate/100,000

Age-standardized death rate/100,000

*Data for Germany are 1999 and 2006.
Nolte, E. McKee, C.M. In amenable mortality — deaths avoidable through healthcare — progress in the U.S. lags that of three European countries. *Health Affairs*. 2012; 31: 92114-2122.

Figure 7: Amenable mortality

The impact of patient expectations and healthcare consumerism

Whenever one is ill or injured, there is an understandable high expectation that the best care will be available and that everything that can be done will be done. While this is likely a universal human desire, or even an expectation, it is particularly true in the American tradition and culture. In addition, as exemplified during the capitation experiment during the 1990s, patients also have high expectations when it comes to choice. They also understandably have high expectations for a caring provider. Survey data and experience suggest patients value their relationship with a trusted clinical advisor more than any other element in healthcare delivery.

It is unlikely these expectations will change in the future. However, as healthcare costs increase and patients are increasingly expected to share a greater portion of the cost burden, when and how these expectations are met is likely to evolve.

As patients become "customers," they are increasingly likely to take charge, and become more attuned to and knowledgeable regarding issues ranging from outcomes and safety rates to increasing insurance deductibles and co-pays. They will pay attention to the costs of diagnostic studies and treatments, and to the nuances of regulatory changes and healthcare reform. Financial insecurity, high unemployment, evaporating assets and savings, and increasing healthcare cost burdens will only add momentum to these trends. Enhanced knowledge will almost certainly result in profound changes to the way patients view and interact with healthcare providers.

Understanding these shifts in patient expectations and how their behaviors are likely to change will be an important step in coming years. Healthcare providers need to be aware of these changes and know how to measure and address them. Recognizing and adapting to these changes will impact everything from patient satisfaction to clinical outcomes, patient flow, models of care that are more patient centric and ambulatory centric, reimbursement, and legal liability risks, making healthcare providers more competitive and less vulnerable.

Meeting patient expectations is more than accommodation — it is risk management because happy patients do not sue. It keeps providers competitive and results in improved clinical care. Good patient experiences lead to better outlooks, improved outcomes, and an enhanced sense of security and wellbeing.

The role of variation in clinical practice

Jack Wennberg, MD, and other health service researchers have documented extensive variation in the delivery of healthcare in many parts of the world. Information on practice variation is important for examining the relationships between policy decisions and clinical decisions. Variation differences also raises important questions concerning the efficiency and effectiveness of healthcare. Variations in healthcare delivery and utilization can indicate potential opportunities to reduce costs and improve the value of healthcare delivery without compromising patient care.

Variations in healthcare spending across the United States have been well documented by Dr. Wennberg as well as other federal and state agencies. The National Health Expenditure data show total per capita healthcare spending ranging from $4,000 in Utah to $6,700 in Massachusetts.[13] Spending variations across smaller geographic units have also been documented using Medicare data. County-by-county analyses by the National

Center for Policy Analysis show Medicare per capita spending in 2008 varied from just over $5,000 in Nobles County, Minnesota, to $8,500 in Rice County, Kansas.[14] Similarly, researchers with the Dartmouth Atlas Project found that among 306 hospital referral regions, Medicare spending per patient ranged from more than $16,000 in some areas to less than $6,000 in others.[15]

Policymakers want to know why healthcare spending is higher in some areas than in others. More specifically, they want to know if there are some efficiencies in low-spending areas that could be replicated in higher-spending areas, thus reducing healthcare costs overall.

In evaluating practice variation, clinical care can be grouped into three categories with different implications for patients, clinicians and policymakers:

- Effective care is defined as interventions for which the benefits far outweigh the risks. In this case the right rate of treatment is 100 percent of patients defined by evidence-based guidelines to be in need, and unwarranted variation is generally a matter of underuse.

- Preference-sensitive care is when more than one generally accepted treatment option is available, such as elective surgery. Here, the right rate should depend on informed patient choice, but treatment rates can vary extensively because of differences in professional opinion.

- Supply-sensitive care comprises clinical activities such as doctor visits, diagnostic tests and hospital admissions, for which the frequency of use relates to the capacity of the local healthcare system. Among older Americans, most of these services are used in caring for chronic illness. However, regions with high rates of use of supply-sensitive care do not have better overall outcomes as measured by mortality and indicators of the quality of care, suggesting that the problem in the U.S. is overuse of this category of care.

Due to unique patient and/or care-setting characteristics, there will always be a degree of appropriate variation in the practice of medicine, even for patients with the same diagnoses. It is clear, however, that through the use of evidence-based and data-based approaches to clinical decision-making, hospitals and other providers across the country can do much more to reduce inappropriate or unwarranted variation.

Inappropriate variation in clinical practice occurs when non-evidence-based care is provided, or when lacking widely accepted evidence-based care, the high level of variation cannot be supported on a quality or outcomes basis. Such care is often driven by nonclinical factors, such as legal, financial, operational (hospital or other care unit processes), or other considerations that providers bring — consciously or unconsciously — to the process of making decisions about how patients are treated. Inappropriate variation can lead to reputational problems for healthcare providers, whether physicians, other clinical staff or affiliated organizations, and often leads to disparate outcomes for patients — either unanticipated or suboptimal outcomes — and higher utilization, costs and waste. The more healthcare providers base their care on good evidence and good data, and the more they standardize their care on best practice, the more they are likely to avoid these pitfalls.

The topic of variation will be discussed in considerably more detail in future chapters.

U.S. healthcare spending

Healthcare spending is the biggest financial issue facing the nation. Spending on healthcare in the United States has been growing precipitously for over three decades and neared $2.6 trillion in 2010, over 10 times the $256 billion spent in 1980, as portrayed in Figure 8.[16]

The rate of growth in recent years has slowed relative to the rate of growth in the late 1990s and early 2000s but is still expected to grow faster than national income over the foreseeable future, as summarized in Figure 9. Addressing this growing burden continues to be a major policy priority at both the national and state level.[16]

In the private sector, employer-based coverage has been a mainstay benefit for decades. Since 2002, premiums for employer-sponsored health coverage for a family have increased by 97 percent, placing increasing cost burdens on employers and workers. An increasing number of U.S. businesses are less

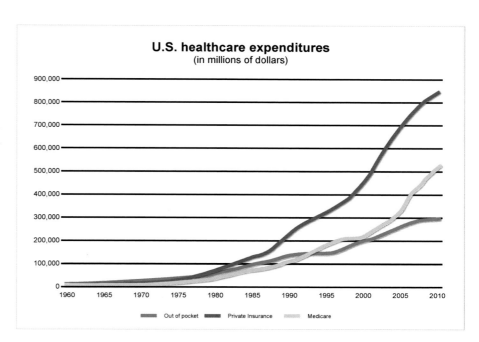

Figure 8: U.S. healthcare expenditures

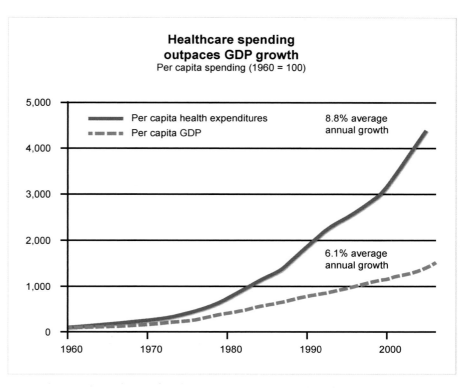

Figure 9: Healthcare spending outpaces GDP growth

competitive globally because of ballooning healthcare costs. Furthermore, the United States has been in a recession or experienced tepid growth for much of the past decade, resulting in higher unemployment and lower incomes for many Americans. U.S. economic woes have heightened the burden of healthcare costs for both individuals and businesses. These conditions have focused even more attention on healthcare spending and affordability.

As a result of these trends, employers are steadily reducing health insurance coverage or eliminating it altogether. An example of this is IBM's recently announced plans to move about 110,000 retirees off its company-sponsored health plan and instead give them a single fixed payment to buy coverage on a health-insurance exchange. This is a clear sign that even big, well-capitalized employers aren't likely to keep providing the once common benefits as medical costs continue to rise. The move, which will affect all IBM retirees once they become eligible for Medicare, will relieve the technology company of the responsibility of managing retirement health-care benefits. In announcing the decision, IBM said the growing cost of care makes its current plan unsustainable without big premium increases. IBM's shift is an indication that health-insurance marketplaces, similar to the public exchanges proposed under the Affordable Care Act, will play a bigger role as companies move coverage down the path taken by many pensions, paying employees and retirees a fixed sum to manage their own care. In the future, increasing premiums and growing marketplace competitiveness will likely lead more employers to reduce or drop coverage.

Many consumers and small employers are also struggling to afford their health insurance premiums. Some employers are not able to offer healthcare coverage at all. For firms with fewer than 10 employees, only 50 percent offered coverage to their workers in 2012. As a result:

> 49 million Americans lacked health insurance in 2011.[17]

> Those consumers with healthcare coverage experienced a 7.2 percent increase in their share of healthcare costs between 2011 and 2012. Healthcare costs for American families in 2012 exceeded $20,000 for the first time.[18]

> Increasingly, Americans are having problems paying for care — 26 percent report they or a family member had problems paying medical bills in the past year. Fifty-eight percent of Americans reported foregoing or delaying medical care in the past year.[19]

In the public sector, Medicare covers the elderly and people with disabilities, and Medicaid provides coverage to low-income families. Enrollment has grown in Medicare with the aging of the baby boomers and in Medicaid due to the recession. This means that total government spending has increased considerably. Escalating healthcare costs also are straining federal and state budgets, hindering the nation's ability to pay for important initiatives needed to address other significant issues. In total, health spending accounted for 17.9 percent of the nation's Gross Domestic Product (GDP) in 2010, as shown in Figure 10.

The U.S. spends far more per capita in both the public and private sectors than any other nation in the world, as illustrated in Figure 11.

These and vast amounts of other spending data make it abundantly clear that change is inevitable. These healthcare spending trends are unsustainable, and in the future they will make change inevitable as private payers, public payers and consumers demand the elimination of waste, better utilization of resources in delivering high-quality and safe care, and new, more efficient care delivery models.

In later chapters of this book, a strong case will be made that high-quality, readily accessible data, sound analytics and effective improvement methodologies are essential to address the quality, safety, access and satisfaction challenges facing healthcare. This is no less true when it comes to addressing healthcare's cost and waste challenges.

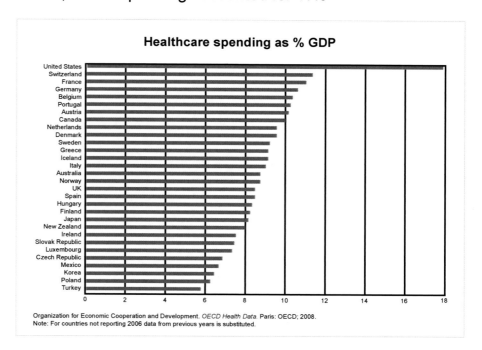

Figure 10: Healthcare spending as a percentage of GDP

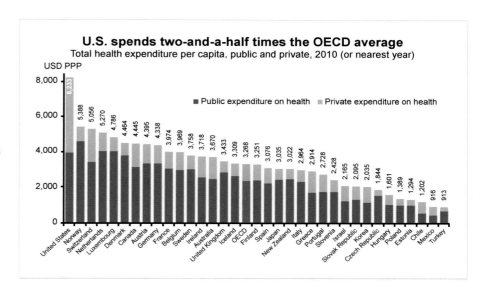

Figure 11: Health expenditures per capita

In the next chapter, we will examine the quality, safety, complexity and human factors that make up the present and future challenges facing healthcare. Following that, in part 2, we will turn our attention to emerging evidence-based and data-driven performance improvement solutions that healthcare providers can implement to address these challenges and more adequately provide patients and communities the care they deserve.

2 PRESENT AND FUTURE CHALLENGES FACING U.S. HEALTHCARE

In the first chapter, we reviewed the historical, cultural, financial, practical, social and traditional forces that define and shape the U.S. healthcare system as it exists today. In this chapter, we provide an overview of the quality, safety and complexity challenges facing healthcare.

Quality challenges facing U.S. healthcare

The IOM has defined the quality of care as "the degree to which health services for individuals and populations increase the likelihood of desired health outcomes and are consistent with current professional knowledge." In its groundbreaking 2001 report, "Crossing the Quality Chasm", the IOM proposed six aims for a quality healthcare system: patient safety, patient-centeredness, effectiveness, efficiency, timeliness and equity.[20] Stated more simply, healthcare quality is getting the right care to the right patient at the right time, every time. It is noteworthy that the IOM framework lists safety as one of their six aims, in essence making patient safety a subset of quality. Some have argued that patient safety is a separate entity, but the fundamental point remains the same. We owe the patients we serve high-quality, safe and effective care. Although many clinicians tend to think of quality as being synonymous with the delivery of evidence-based care, it is noteworthy that the IOM's definition is significantly broader and includes elements that are of particular importance to patients (patient-centeredness and timeliness) and to society (equity).

Although the IOM makes it clear that quality is more than providing care that is supported by science, evidence-based medicine still provides the foundation for much of quality measurement and improvement. For decades, the particular practice experience and style of a senior clinician or a prestigious medical center determined the standard of care. Without discounting the value of experience and mature clinical judgment, the model for determining optimal practice has shifted, driven by an explosion in clinical research over the past two generations. Over the past four decades, the number of randomized clinical trials has grown from fewer than 500 per year in 1970 to 20,000 per year in 2010. This research has helped define "best practices" in many areas of clinical care, ranging from preventive strategies for an elderly woman with diabetes to the treatment of the patient with acute myocardial infarction and cardiogenic shock.

Spending doesn't equal care

Although the U.S. spends more money per person on healthcare than any other nation in the world, there is broad evidence that Americans often do not get the care they need. Preventive care is underutilized, resulting in higher spending on complex, advanced diseases. A Rand study published in 1998 demonstrated that only 50 percent of Americans receive recommended preventative care. Among patients with acute illnesses, only 70 percent received recommended treatments and 30 percent received contraindicated treatments. Patients with chronic diseases such as congestive heart failure, hypertension, ischemic heart disease and diabetes all too often do not receive proven and effective treatments such as drug therapies or self-management services to help them more effectively manage their conditions. In another RAND study, patients with chronic disease received recommended treatments only 60 percent of the time, and 20 percent of the time they received contraindicated treatments.[21, 22] This is true irrespective of one's ability to pay — that is, for insured, uninsured and underinsured Americans. These problems are exacerbated by a lack of coordination of care for patients with chronic diseases.

Yet another RAND study, reported in the New England Journal of Medicine in 2003, concluded that American healthcare gets it right only 54.9 percent of the time.[22] Additional highlights from the study included the following:

- Performance was strikingly similar in all twelve communities studied. Overall quality ranged from 59 percent in Seattle, Washington, to 51 percent in Little Rock, Arkansas. The researchers found the same basic level of performance for chronic, acute and preventive care.

- Quality varied substantially across conditions. For example, people with high blood pressure received about 65 percent of recommended care; persons with alcohol dependence received about 11 percent.

- Quality also varied across communities for the same condition. For example, care for diabetes ranged from 39 percent in Little Rock to 59 percent in Miami. Care for cardiac problems ranged from 52 percent in Indianapolis and Orange County to 70 percent in Syracuse.

- All communities did a better job of preventing chronic disease through screening tests (e.g., measuring blood pressure) and immunizations than in preventing other types of disease, such as sexually transmitted diseases, and in providing other types of preventive care, such as counseling for substance abuse.

- No single community had consistently the highest or lowest performance for all of the chronic conditions. The relative rankings of the communities changed depending on the aspect of care being examined.

- Everyone is at risk for poor care. Race, gender or financial status makes only a small difference in the likelihood of receiving recommended care. For example, women were more likely to receive recommended preventive care, but men receive better-quality care for acute conditions. Previous studies have demonstrated disparities in care for blacks associated with invasive and expensive procedures, such as coronary-artery bypass graft surgery. However, based on the broad RAND measures, which assessed more routine care, blacks were slightly more likely than whites or Hispanics to receive recommended care for chronic conditions, whereas Hispanics were most likely to receive recommended screening.[21]

Reforming to deliver improved quality of care

While many patients often do not receive medically necessary care, others receive care that may be unnecessary, or even harmful. Research has documented tremendous variation in hospital inpatient lengths of stay, visits to specialists, procedures and testing, and costs — not only by different geographic areas of the U.S. but also from hospital to hospital in the same community. This variation has no apparent beneficial impact on the health of the populations being treated. Limited evidence on which treatments and procedures are most effective, the inability to inform providers about the effectiveness of different treatments, and failures to detect and reduce errors further contributes to gaps in the quality and efficiency of care. These issues are particularly relevant to lower-income Americans and to members of diverse ethnic and demographic groups who often face great disparities in health and healthcare.

Reforming our healthcare delivery system to improve the quality and value of care is essential to addressing escalating costs, poor quality and increasing numbers of Americans without health insurance coverage. Reforms should improve access to the right care at the right time in the right setting. They should keep people healthy and prevent common, avoidable complications associated with illnesses to the greatest extent possible. Thoughtfully constructed reforms would support greater access to high-quality, safe and effective care in contrast to the current system, which encourages more tests, procedures and treatments — many of which are at best unnecessary and at worst harmful and costly.

A conceptual framework for evaluating quality of care

In 1966, Avedis Donabedian, a physician and health services researcher, developed a conceptual structure-process-outcome framework for examining health services and evaluating quality of care.[23] His framework has been widely used to measure the quality of care. Donabedian argued that before assessing quality we must come to an agreement regarding how we define it. The definition depends on whether one assesses only the performance of practitioners or also the contributions of patients and of the healthcare system, on how broadly health and responsibility for health are defined, on whether the "maximally" effective or "optimally" effective care is sought, and on whether individual or societal preferences define the optimum. One also needs detailed information regarding the causal linkages among the structural attributes of the settings in which care occurs, the processes of care and the outcomes of care.

According to the Donabedian Model (Figure 12), information about quality of care can be drawn from three categories: structure, process, and outcomes.[23] Structure describes the context in which care is delivered, including hospital buildings, staff, financing and equipment. Process denotes the transactions between patients and providers throughout the delivery of healthcare. Finally, outcomes refer to the effects of healthcare on the health status of patients and populations. While the Donabedian Model has limitations and there are other quality of care frameworks, it continues to be the dominant standard for assessing the quality of healthcare.[23] In recent years, as clinical research has established the link between certain processes and improved outcomes, process measures have often been used as proxies for quality. Examples include measuring whether hospitalized patients with pneumonia received influenza and pneumococcal vaccinations, and measuring glycosylated hemoglobin (hemoglobin A1c) at appropriate intervals in outpatients with diabetes.

Donabedian went on to explore the link between benefits and cost (Figure 13). Imagine you are treating a patient and you are going to spend exactly the same amount of money each day in treating the patient. If you track cost over time (where the X axis is time moving ahead), your cost will go up at a constant rate, as shown in the top graph of Figure 13. As healthcare professionals, we usually try to use the things that work best first. If we use those treatments, we expect the patient to receive a benefit (green line). Eventually, we will exhaust the "first tier" treatments and we will need to turn to "second tier" treatments. As a result, while our costs continue to rise at a constant rate, the

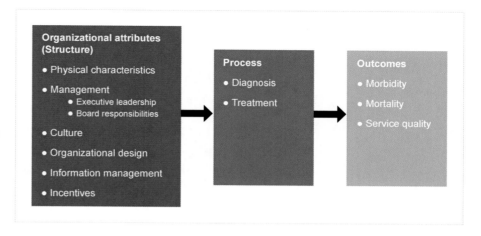

Figure 12: The Donabedian Model of measuring healthcare system performance

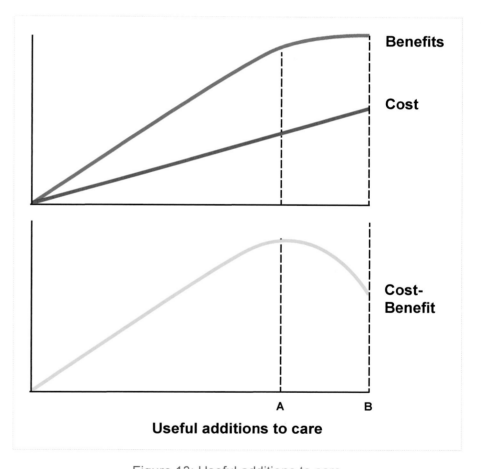

Figure 13: Useful additions to care

benefit will taper off. As you move beyond point A, the benefit will drop off and the inherent risks are likely to rise, leading to a lower cost-benefit, as shown in the lower graph of Figure 13. Ideally, you would push for peak benefit for the patient, which is point B. Donabedian called this a "maximalist" approach. That is, you are seeking maximum benefit for the patient under your care.

Now, imagine that we don't think of just one patient at a time, but instead we are tasked with care delivery for a population. In addition, let's accept reality: we have a finite number of resources at our disposal. In that situation, we are likely going to want to pay attention to a cost-benefit curve. This is the slope of the green line (benefits) divided by the slope of the red line (cost). Donabedian pointed out that if you want maximum benefit across a population you want to be at the peak of the cost-benefit curve (point A on the lower graph in Figure 13). Donabedian called this an "optimalist" approach because the focus is achieving the maximum benefit across a population, rather than for an individual patient. If we are going to spend more treatment money, we would prefer to find a patient located before point A, where the slope of the curve is still going up, indicating that patient will get more benefit than a patient beyond point A. Using this population perspective, it is apparent that there is a difference when focusing on the whole (population) rather than on an individual patient.

Donabedian's intent was to foster a discussion about the ethics of patient care, particularly patient benefit as opposed to population benefit. If we are talking about a population, we have a responsibility to ask patients as a group how much healthcare they want to buy at what benefit and cost. Donabedian argued this was not a care provider's decision. Instead, it was the decision of the population of patients — that is, society. In such situations, care providers have an obligation to help society understand the trade-offs.

Causes of practice variation

Practice variance can occur in the Donabedian Model categories of process and outcomes. Inappropriate variation is a known cause of poor quality and outcomes. Based on a detailed review of the literature, Dr. Brent James and colleagues have identified a long list of reasons for inappropriate practice variation.[24] Here are the top four on the list:

> An increasingly complex healthcare environment. Over the last 50 years, we have witnessed huge changes in how care is delivered, with massive growth in complexity. In the 1950s, physicians had a small number of medications to choose from. Now, there are more than 10,000 prescription drugs and biologicals — and 300,000 over-the-counter products — available in the United States.[25] There have been equally profound changes in care delivery options and environments, including modern imaging techniques, highly sophisticated intensive

care units and surgical suites, catheter-based procedures, transplant services, minimally invasive techniques, and a host of other complicated options. Under the current system, care providers are being overwhelmed with complexity. As stated by David Eddy, MD, "The complexity of modern American medicine exceeds the capacity of the unaided human mind."

⊘ Exponentially increasing medical knowledge. In 1998, Mark Chassin published an article tracking the publication of randomly controlled trials (RCTs) between 1966 and 1995.[26] One look at Figure 14 and it is apparent that there has been an explosion in the production of published trials. The number of randomized clinical trials had grown to over 20,000 per year in 2010.

In 2004, the U.S. National Library of Medicine added almost 11,000 new articles per week to its online archives.[27] That represented only about 40 percent of all articles published worldwide in biomedical and clinical journals. In 2009, it was estimated that this rate of production had grown to one article every 1.29 minutes. Furthermore, Shaneyfelt estimated in 2001 that approximately three to four years after board

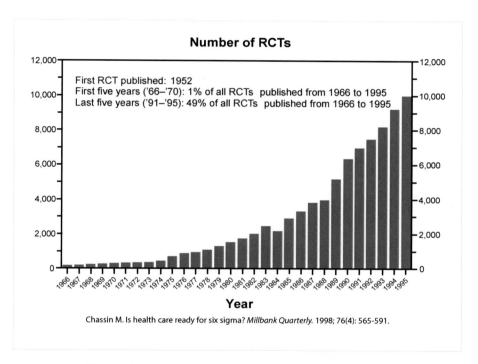

Chassin M. Is health care ready for six sigma? *Millbank Quarterly.* 1998; 76(4): 565-591.

Figure 14: Publication of randomly controlled trials

certification, general internist and internal medicine subspecialists begin to show "significant declines in medical knowledge."[28] He estimated that 15 years after initial board certification approximately 68 percent of internists would not pass the American Board of Internal Medicine certification exam. He went on to estimate that to maintain current knowledge, a general internist would need to read 20 articles a day, 365 days a year. Clearly, maintaining current knowledge has become a near impossible task for all clinicians.

⊘ Lack of valid clinical knowledge (inadequate evidence for what we do). There have been three published studies looking at the percentage of clinical care that is based on published scientific research.[29, 30, 31] These studies have concluded that only between 10 percent and 20 percent of routine medical practice has a basis in scientific research. Thus, much of what we do in routine clinical practice is based on tradition or opinion. That doesn't necessarily mean it is wrong, as much of it has likely been shown to work over time. However, it does suggest that healthcare delivery organizations should use their own data to determine the efficacy of clinical practice and to determine how to improve it over time. This implies the need to create a data-driven continuous learning environment. We will discuss that topic in greater detail in future chapters.

> Overreliance on subjective judgment. Dr. David Eddy and others have demonstrated that the beliefs of experts with respect to a given clinical condition can vary over a very wide range and that subjective evaluation is notoriously poor across groups over time.[32] For example, a group of experts was asked what overall reduction in colon cancer incidence and mortality could be expected from the routine use of fecal occult blood testing and flexible sigmoidoscopy. The answers varied between near 0 percent and over 90 percent, with a completely random distribution.[32] Dr. Eddy's intent was not to disparage the value of a specialist's advice — it is valuable. Rather, it was to demonstrate that even the busiest specialist is dealing with a sample size that is too small to draw general conclusions. These findings and others have caused Dr. Eddy to conclude, "You can find a physician who honestly believes — and will testify in court to — anything you want."

The underlying fragmentation of the healthcare system also contributes to poor quality. It impedes the flow and integration of the data necessary for healthcare providers to provide the best possible care. This fragmentation is not surprising given that healthcare providers do not have the payment support, incentives or other tools they need to communicate and work together effectively to improve patient care.

Challenges related to patient safety

In its seminal report, "To Err Is Human: Building a Safer Health System", the IOM conservatively estimated that as many as 44,000 to 98,000 Americans die each year as a result of preventable medical error.[33] While many articles on the topic of patient safety had been published prior to this, the IOM report crystallized and energized the discussion and debate regarding patient safety and harm, and launched the rapidly evolving and highly dynamic field of patient safety. Over the past decade, much progress has been made in our understanding of patient safety, and considerable progress has been made in reducing harm. This subsection will review the current state of our knowledge. While the goal is for this to be a reasonable review of patient safety, the reader is strongly encouraged to read "Understanding Patient Safety" by Robert Wachter, MD (second edition, 2012).[34] This well researched, comprehensive and highly readable text is a must read for anyone interested in improving patient care.

The IOM report on harm has proven to be groundbreaking from many different perspectives, but the single and most influential fact emanating from the report was the number of deaths resulting from preventable patient harm. This number justifiably garnered significant attention and generated a long-overdue debate. This is not surprising given that it represents the rough equivalent of a fully loaded Boeing 747 crashing every day of the year! One can only imagine the attention an aviation disaster of this magnitude would generate among the public. Yet the number dying from preventable patient harm in U.S. hospitals had gone largely unnoticed prior to the IOM report.

In the early months following the publication of the report, some wanted to argue the accuracy of the number, but even if the numbers are off by half, this obviously still represents an unacceptable rate of harm (it is noteworthy that some knowledgeable experts have estimated that the range of deaths from avoidable harm is actually higher). Even if you only accept the lower estimate in the IOM range, medical error is still the ninth leading cause of death in the United States. It surpasses deaths due to motor vehicle accidents, chronic liver disease, alcohol-induced and drug-induced deaths (combined), and a variety of cancers, including breast, stomach and prostate.[35] While staggering, these estimates of death due to harm only begin to scratch the surface of the problem, as they fail to measure the full range of adverse events stemming from injuries not resulting in death.[33, 36, 37]

Regardless of how one measures it, medical error is an important indicator of quality in healthcare, reflecting the overuse, underuse and misuse of health services.[20, 33, 38] Particularly in the case of misuse, preventable harm from medical treatment compromises patient safety and may result in injury or death. Variations in clinical care also undermine patient trust in the healthcare system.[39] In the end, medical error and harm prevent healthcare providers from achieving their potential in service to patients. The social cost of harm is enormous, estimated to be between $29 and $38 billion per year, with about $17 billion of those costs associated with preventable errors.[40, 41]

The IOM and many patient safety experts stress that most medical errors reflect system errors rather than individual misconduct or negligence.[33] This is an important distinction because engaging clinicians in reducing harm requires that we acknowledge that the problem is not fundamentally a "bad apple" problem. As Dr. Wachter said in his book, "Internal Bleeding: The Truth Behind America's Epidemic of Medical Mistakes":

> *Decades of research, mostly from outside healthcare, has confirmed our own medical experience: Most errors are made by good but fallible people working in dysfunctional systems, which means that making care safer depends on buttressing the system to prevent or catch*

the inevitable lapses of mortals. This logical approach is common in other complex, high-tech industries, but it has been woefully ignored in medicine. Instead, we have steadfastly clung to the view that an error is a moral failure by an individual, a posture that has left patients feeling angry and ready to blame, and providers feeling guilty and demoralized. Most importantly, it hasn't done a damn thing to make healthcare safer.[42]

While it is true that most preventable harm is not a "bad apple" problem, Drs. Wachter and Peter Provonost have appropriately argued that we need to balance no blame and professional accountability.[43] That is, we need to acknowledge that there are indeed some "bad apples."

Reducing avoidable patient harm and advancing patient safety will require a comprehensive, intricate and thoughtful approach. To quote Dr. Wachter from the introduction to the second edition of his book:

> Decades of research, mostly from outside healthcare, has confirmed our own medical experience: Most errors are made by good but fallible people working in a dysfunctional a system, which means that making care safer depends on buttressing the system to prevent or catch the inevitable lapses of mortals.
>
> — Dr. Robert Wachter

To keep patients safe will take a uniquely interdisciplinary effort, one in which doctors, nurses, pharmacists, and administrators forge new types of relationships. It will demand that we look to other industries for good ideas, while recognizing that caring for patients is different enough from other human endeavors that thoughtful adaptation is critical. It will require that we tamp down our traditionally rigid hierarchies, without forgetting the importance of leadership or compromising crucial lines of authority. It will take additional resources, although investments in safety may well pay off in new efficiencies, lower provider turnover, and fewer expensive complications. It will require a thoughtful embrace of this new notion of systems thinking, while recognizing the absolute importance of the well-trained and committed caregiver.

As this quote indicates, there has been a concerted effort over the last decade to shift the focus of patient safety from a "blame and shame" game to a systems thinking approach. The fact is fallible humans will always be prone to error, particularly in increasingly complex environments like healthcare. Reducing harm and making care safer depends on creating systems in all care environments that anticipate errors and either prevent them or catch them before they cause harm. This approach has produced remarkable safety records in other industries, including aviation, and we are overdue in applying it to healthcare.

Avoidable error and harm categories

Safety experts including Lucian Leape, Robert Wachter, Peter Pronovost and others have organized the causes of avoidable errors and harm into the following logical categories:[34]

- Medication errors. Adverse drug events (ADEs) are a significant source of patient harm. The medication delivery process is enormously complex. On the inpatient side alone, it generally represents dozens of steps, and it is only marginally less complicated in the ambulatory environment. Taken appropriately, the thousands of medications available in clinical care today offer huge advantages to patients. Still, the thousands of available drug options and their complicated interaction with human physiology and each other leads to a significant incidence of near misses (5 to 10 percent) and actual adverse drug events (5 percent) in hospitalized patients.[44]

  The incidence of ADEs is significantly higher for high-risk medications like insulin, warfarin or heparin.[45] In addition to patient harm, the cost of preventable medication errors in hospitalized patients in the U.S. is substantial, estimated at $16.4 billion annually.[46] In the ambulatory environment, the incidence of harm and the costs are even higher.[47]

  Multiple solutions are required to address the issue of adverse drug events. These include several well-implemented technological solutions: computerized physician order entry (CPOE), computerized decision support, bar code medication administration, and radio-frequency identification (RFID) systems. It will also require addressing a number of process issues, including standardization, vigilance with respect to the "Five Rights" (right patient, right route, right dose, right time and right drug), double checks, preventing interruptions and distractions, removal of high-risk medications from certain areas, optimizing the role of clinical pharmacists, addressing the issue of look-alike and sound-alike medications, and implementing effective medication reconciliation processes, particularly at hand-off points.

- Surgical errors. There are over 20 million surgeries annually in the U.S. In recent years, a number of advances have resulted in significant improvements in the safety of surgery and anesthesia and reductions in harm and death.[48] Still, a number of surgical safety challenges persist. These include persistent anesthesia-related complications, wrong-site surgeries, wrong patient surgeries, retained foreign bodies and surgical fires. One study indicated that 3 percent of inpatients who underwent surgery suffered an adverse event, and half of these were preventable.[49] Studies have also shown that there is a strong relationship between volume and safety. That is, surgeons need to perform any given surgery a certain number of times to attain a level of skill required to minimize adverse surgical events. Addressing surgical safety will require a number of measures, including widespread adoption of safety principles already largely implemented by anesthesiologists (e.g., systems thinking, human factors engineering, learning from mistakes, standardization and comprehensively applying the "Universal Protocols" — including site signing and time outs), along with teamwork training, checklists and the use of best practices for minimizing retained foreign bodies and avoiding surgical fires.

> **Diagnostic errors.** While they have received less emphasis, diagnostic errors are relatively common. For example, in the study that served as the basis for the IOM's estimate of 44,000 to 98,000 annual deaths from preventable errors, 17 percent of the deaths were attributed to diagnostic errors.[50] Furthermore, autopsy studies have demonstrated that 1 in 10 patients suffer a major antemortem error.[51] Addressing this problem will require a number of measures, including avoiding fatigue, avoiding overreliance on past experience, improved training in cognitive reasoning and computerized decision support systems.

> **Person-machine interface errors (human factors engineering).** Human factors engineering is an applied science of systems design that is concerned with the interplay between humans, machines and their work environments. Its goal is to assure that devices, systems and working environments are designed to minimize the likelihood of error and optimize safety. As one of its central tenets, the field recognizes that humans are fallible — they often overestimate their abilities and underestimate their limitations. This is particularly important in the increasingly complex healthcare environment, where fallible care providers are being overwhelmed by increasing complexity.

Many complex care environments have little or no support from modern technology for care providers, and in those that do have such support the devices often have poorly designed user interfaces that are difficult and even dangerous to use.[52, 53] Human factors engineers strive to understand the strengths and weaknesses of human physical and mental abilities. They use that information to design safer devices, systems and environments. Thoughtful application of human factors engineering principles can assist humans dealing with complex care environments and help prevent errors at the person–machine interface.

> **Errors at transitions of care (handoff errors).** Transitions of care between care environments and care providers are common in clinical care. These handoffs are a common source of patient harm. One study demonstrated that 12 percent of patients experienced preventable adverse events after hospital discharge, most commonly

medication errors.[54] Because they are so common, healthcare provider organizations increasingly are focusing on this type of harm.

Policymakers are also paying more attention to this type of harm. In 2006, the Joint Commission issued a National Patient Safety Goal that requires healthcare organizations to implement a standardized approach to handoff communications including an opportunity to ask and respond to questions. Because of studies showing very high 30-day readmission rates in Medicare patients (20 percent overall, nearly 30 percent in patients with heart failure), Medicare began penalizing hospitals with high readmission rates in 2012.[55] All of this attention has stimulated a growing body of research focused on handoffs and transitions. This research is providing a deeper understanding of best practices, which have both structural and interpersonal components. These practices include standardized communication protocols (including "read backs") and more interoperable information systems.

> Teamwork and communication errors. Medicine is fundamentally a team sport. There is an overwhelming amount of evidence that the quality of teamwork often determines whether patients receive appropriate care promptly and safely. There are many clinical examples of this, including the management of a cardiac arrest (a so-called "code blue"), a serious trauma case, a complicated surgery, the delivery of a compromised infant or the treatment of an immune-compromised patient in isolation.

While the importance of teamwork is widely accepted, the evidence that it exists and that team members feel free to speak up if they see unsafe conditions is not strong.[56] Over the last three decades, the aviation industry has learned the importance of teamwork and implemented state-of-the-art teamwork concepts which have had a dramatic impact on safety performance (Figure 15).[57] Healthcare patient safety advocates have appropriately turned to the aviation industry to adapt their teamwork concepts to clinical care.

In addition, the JCAHO sentinel event program has provided evidence that communication problems are the most

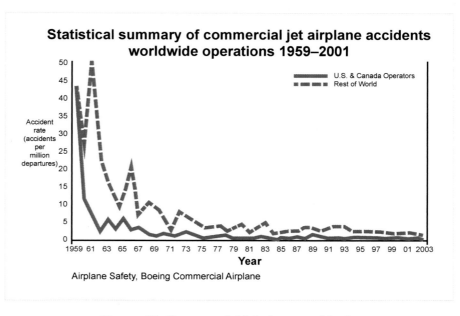

Figure 15: Commercial jet plane accidents

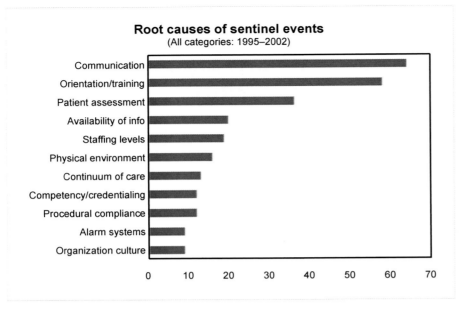

Root causes of sentinel events
(All categories: 1995–2002)

Figure 16: Root cause of sentinel events

common root cause of serious medical errors, as shown in Figure 16.[58]

Well-functioning healthcare teams should employ appropriate authority gradients that allow people to speak up, utilize aviation's crew resource training communication model (CRM), use effective methods of reviewing and updating information on individual patients, employ accepted strategies to improve communications including SBAR (Situation, Background, Assessment and Recommendation) and so-called "CUS words" (I am Concerned, I am Uncomfortable and I feel it is a Safety issue) to express escalating levels of concern, and constantly maintain situational awareness.

> Healthcare-associated infections (HAIs). Healthcare-associated infections (HAI) are infections that people acquire in a healthcare setting while they are receiving treatment for another condition. HAIs can be acquired anywhere healthcare is delivered, including inpatient acute care hospitals, outpatient settings such as ambulatory surgical centers and end-stage renal disease facilities, and long-term care facilities such as nursing homes and rehabilitation centers. HAIs may be caused by any infectious agent, including bacteria, fungi and viruses, as well as other less common types of pathogens.

These infections are associated with a variety of risk factors, including:

> Use of indwelling medical devices such as bloodstream, endotracheal and urinary catheters

> Surgical procedures

> Injections

> Contamination of the healthcare environment

> Transmission of communicable diseases between patients and healthcare workers

> Overuse or improper use of antibiotics

HAIs are a significant cause of morbidity and mortality. The CDC estimates that 1 in 20 hospitalized patients will develop an HAI, that they are responsible for about 100,000 deaths per year in U.S. hospitals alone and that HAIs are responsible for $30 to $40 billion in costs.[59] In addition, HAIs can have devastating emotional, medical and legal consequences.

The following list covers the majority of HAIs:

> Catheter-associated urinary tract infections

> Surgical site infections

> Bloodstream infections (including central line-associated infections)

> Pneumonia (including ventilator-associated pneumonia)

> Methicillin-resistant Staph aureus infections (MRSA)

> *C. difficile* infection

As they are to other common sources of harm, federal policymakers are paying attention to HAIs. The U.S. Department of Health and Human Services (HHS) has identified the reduction of HAIs as an agency priority goal for the department. HHS committed to reducing the national rate of HAIs by demonstrating significant, quantitative and measurable reductions in hospital-acquired central line-associated bloodstream infections and catheter-associated urinary tract infections by no later than September 30, 2013. The final results of this program are yet to be published.

By using a variety of well-tested policies and procedures, there is encouraging evidence that healthcare organizations can significantly decrease the frequency of HAIs.[60, 61, 62]

◉ Other sources of errors. There are a variety of other sources of significant patient harm in clinical care. These include patient falls, altered mental status (often due to over sedation), pressure ulcers and venous thromboembolism, harm related to inadequate staffing ratios, harm resulting from nonstandardization, errors due to lack of redundant systems, harm resulting from inadequate provider training, harm caused by caregiver stress and fatigue, etc.

The role of information technology and measurement in safety

Advanced information technology is playing an increasingly important role in patient safety. Technologies involved include Electronic Health Records (EHRs), CPOE, clinical decision support systems, IT systems designed to improve diagnostic accuracy, analytical systems, bar coding, RFID, smart intravenous pumps and automated drug dispensing systems. It is important to note that skill is required to implement these systems in a manner that promotes safety while not increasing the rate of harm.

Measuring errors and rates of harm can be a difficult process. Traditionally, measuring systems have depended on voluntary reporting, but for a variety of reasons, it is clear that these approaches significantly underestimate errors and harm. Other approaches, such as patient safety indicators drawn from administrative datasets, can be overly sensitive and therefore need to be augmented by detailed chart reviews.

Over the past decade, the use of trigger tools has emerged as a favored method to measure the incidence of adverse events in a healthcare organization. The most widely used of these is the Global Trigger Tool (GTT). Initially developed by David Classen, MD, and others, the GTT has been adopted and promoted by the Institute for Healthcare Improvement (IHI). The theory behind trigger tools is that some errors in care will produce a response that can be tracked, providing clues to possible adverse events. For example, the use of Narcan might indicate over sedation with a narcotic, and the use of Benadryl may indicate an allergic reaction. In most organizations, use of the GTT is fairly labor intensive, but some organizations have made progress in automating the process.

Several studies have looked at the GTT as a way to assess the state of patient safety with somewhat concerning conclusions. One study tracked the rate of adverse events in nine hospitals over five years and found no significant improvement in harm rates despite major efforts to improve patient safety.[63] A study by the Office of Inspector General (OIG) found one in eight Medicare inpatients experienced significant adverse events.[64] Another study used the GTT to demonstrate that one in three hospitalized patients experienced an adverse event of some kind.[65]

This concludes the high-level overview of patient safety. As mentioned at the outset, this overview is not designed to provide the level of detailed knowledge required for healthcare leaders to adequately implement a comprehensive patient safety program. Again, the reader is encouraged to read Dr. Wachter's excellent book on the subject, "Understanding Patient Safety" (second edition, 2012).[34]

Viewing healthcare as a complex adaptive system

Most would agree that healthcare is becoming overwhelmingly complex. In the 1960s, the typical general practitioner practiced in a privately owned office with minimal staff, subscribed to one or two journals, periodically engaged a specialist when necessary, conducted patient rounds in the hospital and did roughly an hour's worth of paperwork a week. Specialists were completely independent, practiced primarily in the hospital, focused principally on a particular body system, were in total control of their practice and interacted with administrators only when they needed some type of support (e.g., the purchase of new equipment).

Those days are essentially gone. As thousands of new drug therapies, sophisticated new forms of diagnosis and treatment, the need for computerization, demands for integrated care, rising demands for data-driven quality outcomes, increasing costs, growing legal liabilities, complex new regulations and a host of other complex, interrelated forces entered the scene, the complexity of clinical care grew exponentially. With these changes, the practice of care has become stressful and often times overwhelming for clinicians and non-clinicians: individual providers, nurses, general practitioners, specialists, administrators and senior executives.

Healthcare organizations are increasingly being viewed as complex adaptive systems. A complex adaptive system is a collection of individual entities that have the ability to act in ways that are not always totally predictable. Furthermore, the entity's actions are interconnected: one entity's actions can sometimes change the context for the other entities, and thereby impact the other entity's actions in unpredictable ways. Examples of complex adaptive systems include the environment, the immune system, the stock market, a colony of insects, world financial markets and families.

Complexity science is the study of complex adaptive systems, the relationships within them, how they are sustained, how they self-organize and how outcomes result. Complexity science is increasingly being applied to healthcare for the reasons outlined above and it offers significant advantages for providers who are trying to understand and manage the growing complexity of healthcare. For those who would like to learn more about healthcare as a complex adaptive system, please read Appendix A.

In conclusion

In part 1, we examined the historical, financial, cultural, quality, safety and complexity factors that characterize healthcare today. In part 2, we will review the emerging concepts and methods that will enable healthcare providers to adapt and succeed in a rapidly changing and increasingly complex future.

PART TWO: LAYING THE FOUNDATION FOR IMPROVEMENT AND SUSTAINABLE CHANGE

Introduction

In part 1 we examined the historical, cultural, financial and social forces that have defined and shaped the healthcare system and the current dynamics that are irreversibly driving the need for change. The purpose of part 2 is to provide a review of emerging concepts and methods that will allow healthcare organizations to adapt to a rapidly changing future. This portion of the book will focus on the quality improvement concepts and tools that organizations need to consider to successfully address the challenges facing healthcare and successfully ride the wave of transformation currently sweeping through our industry.

Over the past decade, it has been my good fortune to encounter many clinicians and healthcare operational leaders across the U.S. In these encounters, two trends have become apparent. First, many of the discussions are increasingly dominated by a common theme — tight budgets and cost cutting. Second, it has been troubling to see many clinicians who represent some of the smartest, best-trained, highly motivated and passionate people I have ever met becoming progressively cynical and disengaged and distancing themselves from important healthcare reform debates.

No doubt there is a need to control costs. But in this focus on cost cutting, are we forgetting the patient? Many countries are struggling with healthcare costs. Healthcare costs are a major part of the national budgets for most industrialized countries, and costs do need to be managed more effectively. Based on this need, it is not surprising that many national reforms are focused on controlling the growth of healthcare costs. The United States is no exception to this trend.

At the same time, healthcare also faces many quality and safety issues. These issues are as equally important to patients as the cost of healthcare. In healthcare, the agents of change are the clinicians who provide patient care. One thing clinicians really care about is the quality of care they deliver to the patients they serve. Like many other professionals, clinicians tend to be competitive. They want to believe they are exceeding the standards for performance, and they think they are committed to continuously improving. Yet, while clinicians really want to believe they are the best, most do not really know if this is true. Clinicians often lack the ability to actually measure the quality of care their patients receive or the outcomes they achieve. As a result, they don't always know what is best for the patient, nor can they learn because they don't have quality and outcomes data.

> When clinicians work together, they can agree on what quality is and start measuring their performance. They can share and debate the data and identify what works best. In the process, everyone can learn from the experience. This is continuous improvement.

A growing number of clinicians are discovering that debating proven practices and choosing the most successful practices based on data is enhancing their professional experience and patient outcomes. Continuous improvement can be rewarding and fun, and it is certainly in line with professional values. But this requires data and a willingness to discover the tested practices that work best. When clinicians work together, they can agree on what quality is and start measuring their performance. They can share and debate the data and identify what works best. In the process, everyone can learn from the experience. This is continuous improvement.

Using data and analysis to drive continuous improvement is exciting, but there's even more good news. If you look at the cost side of the equation, it turns out that those who focus on quality frequently have the lowest costs. Published studies based on Dr. Jack Wennberg's data indicate that if all U.S. healthcare providers operated at the same level as the top 10 percent of performers, it would vastly improve care and lower Medicare costs by about 20 percent.[66] Furthermore, the quality of U.S. healthcare for many diseases is actually below average based on data from the Organization for Economic Co-operation and Development (OECD). If the U.S. healthcare system would focus more on measuring quality and strive to raise quality just to the level of the average OECD data, it would improve care and save the American people $500 billion a year. That represents approximately 20 percent of the annual U.S. healthcare budget.[67]

Most clinicians would agree that these numbers are logical and the potential for savings is exciting, but are they possible to achieve? In order to achieve these savings, a shift towards measuring value in healthcare — that is, not only costs but also the optimized clinical outcomes that actually matter to patients — needs to occur.

This is not just a nice idea. It is actually happening. Groups of innovative clinicians are already forming, identifying evidence-based care practices, measuring outcomes and continuously improving care for the patients they serve. In the process, these clinicians are asking a number of key questions: What is quality? What should we measure? How can we achieve the best outcomes? How can we continuously improve? Disease by disease, they are attacking the medical conditions that afflict humanity, and in the process they are improving the value of care being delivered to patients.

> " By measuring value in healthcare we will understand that clinicians are generally not the problem. Instead, they are an important part of the solution. Measuring value in healthcare will bring about a revolution. This will make Sir William Osler and the other great clinical innovators who revolutionized healthcare a century ago smile in their graves. "

Based on personal experience, I can tell you that every time a group of clinicians embarks on this quest, there is enormous energy in the room. This is because the reform debate has suddenly shifted to what matters most to both clinicians and patients: the value of care that patients are receiving. The future will mandate that healthcare organizations are managed based on what matters to patients, the quality of care they receive. In the process, we can — and will — manage costs.

By measuring value in healthcare we will understand that clinicians are generally not the problem. Instead, they are an important part of the solution. Measuring value in healthcare will bring about a revolution. This will make

Sir William Osler and the other great clinical innovators who revolutionized healthcare a century ago smile in their graves.

In the future, all healthcare delivery organizations will need to transform themselves in order to meet the quality, safety and cost challenges confronting healthcare. In this process, they will need to implement value and clinician engagement strategies that allow them to optimize clinical outcomes and provide care as efficiently as possible. With that in mind, this part of the book will focus on quality improvement concepts and tools that organizations need to consider so they can successfully address the challenges facing healthcare and successfully ride the wave of transformation that is sweeping across the industry. In particular, we will discuss three systems for effective care delivery to help clinicians understand what is needed to effectively improve care and sustain quality improvements.

It is important for clinical and operational leaders to understand quality and continuous improvement principles and how they can drive improved outcomes across the care delivery system if they are going to survive in the emerging new healthcare world. We will describe the theory behind the principles and concepts and then describe how these are applied through practical examples. For example, we will explain the principles around eliminating variation, and then, using the Pareto principle (i.e., 80/20 rule), we will demonstrate how improvement teams can measure variation and prioritize opportunities based on significant variation in clinical processes.

By the end of part 2, you should understand what the following three systems are and how they can be used to help improve care: analytic system, deployment system and content system. The analytic system provides the data and analysis; the deployment system is used to organize work and teams; the content system focuses on how evidence and knowledge are gathered, evaluated and integrated into care delivery.

3 A SYSTEMATIC APPROACH TO SUSTAINABLE QUALITY IMPROVEMENT

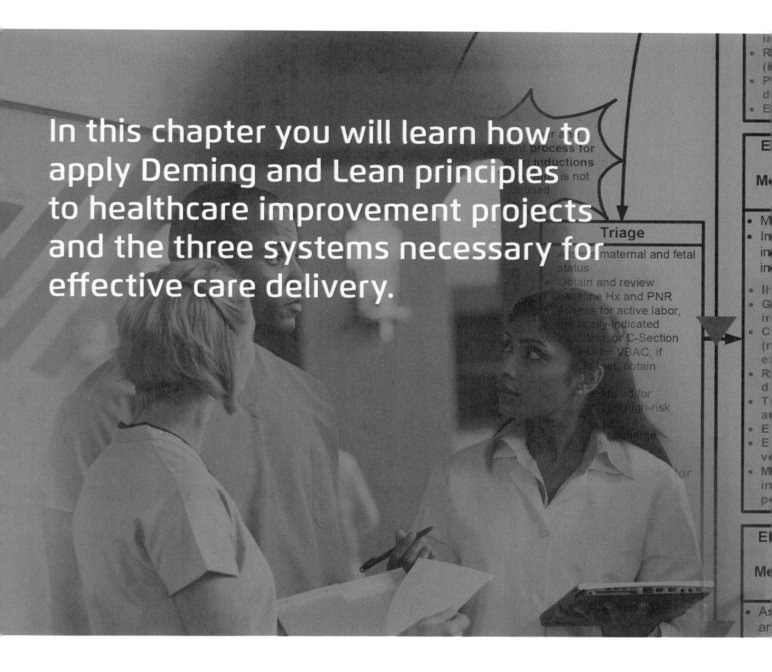

In this chapter you will learn how to apply Deming and Lean principles to healthcare improvement projects and the three systems necessary for effective care delivery.

Let's start with a question. Why do we often see advertisements like the one on the top of Figure 17, but never see advertisements like the one on the bottom? When a friend or family member experiences an illness or injury,

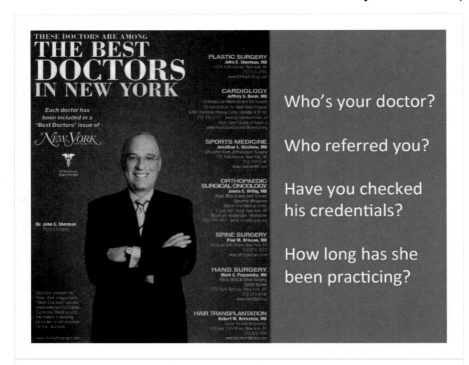

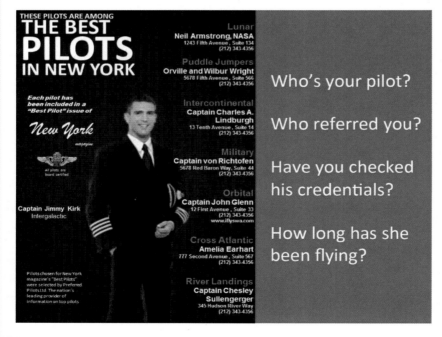

Figure 17: Standardizing healthcare

have you found yourself asking the questions shown in Figure 17 about the physicians who are managing the care of you or your loved ones? You probably have. Yet, why don't we ask similar questions about airline pilots? In general, people feel confident boarding a plane, regardless of who their pilot is. Why is that? And why isn't the same true when picking or visiting a doctor?

People ask these questions because they believe there are big differences between doctors, and they are right. As discussed in chapter 1, Dr. Wennberg, a leading researcher on variation in healthcare, found that geography strongly affects what treatment a patient receives. In fact, the treatment depends as much on a physician's location as it does on the disease state and severity.

The healthcare industry suffers from a lack of standardization. Healthcare will need to adopt a high degree of standardization and move toward a true system of production, as the airline and many other industries have done, in order to deal with the quality, safety and cost challenges facing the industry. Variations in care delivery and utilization often indicate potential opportunities to reduce costs and improve the value of healthcare delivery without negatively compromising the quality of care a patient receives.

We have supplier-induced demand. It's a Field of Dreams mentality — build it and they will come. Buy equipment and then make sure to use it. Add a wing to a hospital and fill the beds. And if a patient is terminal, approach it like Star Trek's Captain Kirk, who famously shouted, "Do something, Bones. She's dying." Better yet, do everything. If there's any chance something might work, try it. All of these practices contribute to high variation, overutilization and skyrocketing costs in healthcare.

> We have supplier-induced demand. It's a Field of Dreams mentality — build it and they will come. Buy equipment and then make sure to use it. Add a wing to a hospital and fill the beds.

The evolution of methods to manage growing organizational complexity

Humans have been managing work for centuries. Initially, approaches to managing work were fairly simple. However, with the passage of time and concomitant growth in demands for efficient, high-volume production of goods and services, managing organizations, production and work became increasingly complex. With this trend came a parallel growth in the sophistication of organizational structures and approaches to management.

Prior to 1800, commerce was dominated by guilds. A guild is essentially an association of artisans, merchants or others with common expertise who control the practice of their craft by limiting membership through a combination of training requirements and governmentally granted power to determine who can and who cannot be a member of the guild. With the advent of capitalism and free trade in the early 19th century, guilds began a long and slow decline in their influence. However, guilds continue to persist in different forms around the world. For example, professional organizations continue to replicate the guild structure and mentality. Professions such as architecture, engineering, law and medicine continue to mandate various training requirements and lengths of apprenticeship before an individual can gain professional certification to practice in the field. Medical "guilds" include medical boards and medical associations (such as the American Medical Association). Licensure to practice medicine in most states requires specific training, passing tests and many years of low-paid apprenticeship under fairly strenuous working conditions. This approach is not dissimilar to guilds that existed prior to the 19th century.

With the industrialization and modernization of trade and industry in the mid-19th century, guilds faded in influence and the beginning of modern organizations occurred with the rise of the factory system, starting first in the textile industry, where automation and mass production became the cornerstone of productivity. With the advent of these modern organizations, there was a need to define what management was and to determine how best to operationalize it.

The first modern management theory to achieve lasting impact and success was scientific management, an approach largely defined and popularized by Frederick Taylor. Taylor began work at age 18 as an apprentice to a patternmaker and machinist. He later joined a steel company as a laborer, ultimately rising to chief engineer over an eight-year period. During this time, Taylor performed detailed experiments on worker productivity and tested what he called the task system, which eventually evolved into his approach to scientific management. Taylor sought to determine the best way of performing each individual work operation, the time it required (using time and motion studies), the materials needed and the optimal work sequence. In taking this approach, he helped formulate the concept of standardized mass production.

While advocating that managers and workers should cooperate, he also tried to establish a clear division of labor between well-educated management and less-educated employees. Taylor believed that managers were not only superior intellectually to the average employee but that managers had a duty to organize and supervise the work activities of front-line employees. Essentially, he saw workers as naturally lazy cogs in a machine. Taylor proposed that simplifying and optimizing jobs would yield greater productivity. Taylor also believed that workers were motivated by money, so he promoted the idea of a fair day's pay for a fair day's work. Conversely, Taylor believed that a worker who did not achieve enough in a day of work did not deserve as much pay as a worker who achieved more.

Taylor accurately predicted the importance of the system as opposed to the individual worker. As Taylor boldly stated, "In the past, the man has been first. In the future, the system will be first."[68] Taylor's principles were widely adopted and they were massively successful. His influence can be seen in factories, schools, offices and hospitals. That is, in essentially any production environment. The scientific management approach to production essentially supplanted the last vestiges of craft-style production. Using Taylor's methods, organizations were able to significantly reduce the effort required to produce goods and services. This led to a huge shift in how organizations conducted their business. Any company that could not successfully implement Taylor's methods simply went out of business. Taylor's theories also led to major social transformations. For example, they contributed significantly to the emergence of the American middle class.

Beginning in about the 1960s, as the work environment became more complex and demands for efficiency and quality grew exponentially, scientific management began to falter as the optimal way to oversee the production of goods and services.

" Beginning in about the 1960s, as the work environment became more complex and demands for efficiency and quality grew exponentially, scientific management began to falter as the optimal way to oversee the production of goods and services. "

Taylorism promotes the idea that there is one right way to do something. In the face of growing complexity, this view was no longer tenable. Fortunately, new management systems and theories more able to handle complexity were ready to take the place of Taylorism, particularly those proposed by W. Edwards Deming.

Deming was a professor of statistics at New York University's graduate school of business. In 1927, he was introduced to the work of William Shewhart of Bell Laboratories. Shewhart had developed the concept of the statistical control of processes and the statistical process control (SPC) chart. Inspired by Shewhart's ideas, Deming began to apply statistical methods to industrial production and management. Shewhart's idea of common and special causes of variation led directly to Deming developing his new theories of management. Deming recognized that his ideas could be applied not only to manufacturing processes but also to processes by which organizations are led and managed. During World War II, Deming taught his methods to workers engaged in wartime production and helped contribute to the U.S.'s achieving unprecedented levels of production during the war.

Although statistical methods were widely and successfully applied during World War II, they faded into disuse in the U.S. once the war ended. Most organizations were focused on mass-producing products to meet huge worldwide demand following the war. In 1947, Deming was asked by the U.S. Army to help plan for the 1951 Japanese census. While in Japan, his expertise in quality control was recognized and led to an invitation from the Japanese Union of Scientists and Engineers (JUSE) to teach his statistical process control and quality improvement methods in Japan as a part of the Japanese post-war reconstruction effort. Deming's message was straightforward: improving quality would reduce expenses while increasing productivity and market share.

Deming continued to develop his statistical improvement methods and successfully helped the Japanese apply them to all sorts of organizations. Over the subsequent two decades, many Japanese manufacturers applied his techniques widely and experienced unprecedented levels of productivity and quality. The combination of high-quality, yet low-cost goods, created massive worldwide demand for Japanese products. In the 1980s, facing their own issues related to complexity coupled with fierce competitive threats from Japan, U.S. organizations finally began to widely adopt Deming's methods. Eventually, they duplicated the high-quality, low-cost outcomes achieved by Japanese manufacturers.

The two keys to Deming's success were producing what customers' wanted and his recognition that successful efforts toward continuous improvement could be built only on the knowledge of front-line workers. Management needs to put quality improvement into the hands of front-line workers and then provide them the support necessary to achieve success. His approach to quality improvement was process focused and data driven. He recognized that if you couldn't measure it, you couldn't improve it. In Deming's words, "In God we trust; all others must bring data."[69]

Deming's improvement methods were further enhanced with the widespread adoption of Lean production, starting in the 1980s. In 1990, James Womack and others popularized Lean production with the publication of their best-selling book "The Machine That Changed the World."[70] Lean production, or Lean for short, is the production practice that considers the expenditure of resources for any goal other than the creation of value for the customer to be wasteful and a target for elimination. In short, Lean is centered on preserving value with less work. Similar to Deming's methods, Lean recognizes the need to empower front-line workers. The goal of Lean is to use standardized processes to eliminate waste but also allow front-line workers — so-called smart cogs — to adapt to individual customer needs as necessary. It utilizes efficient processes that can deal with complexity, yet also supports mass customization. A classic example is Dell, a world leader in Lean methods. A customer can go to the Dell website and order a personal computer with very detailed individual specifications, and the computer will be efficiently built to exactly those specifications. In fact, Dell's process is so efficient, it often takes longer to ship a Dell PC to a customer than it does to manufacture it. This is Lean production. It allows front-line workers to drive out waste using optimized workflows and standardized processes while also providing room to adapt to individual customer needs. As we will see later, this approach has high applicability to healthcare.

Advancing to a system of production

Figure 18 illustrates the evolution of process management. In the healthcare industry, we still have a craftsmanship mentality to process management. Even the way physicians are trained reflects more of a craftsmanship approach because it relies heavily on whom they shadow during their residency, resulting in inconsistency in expertise

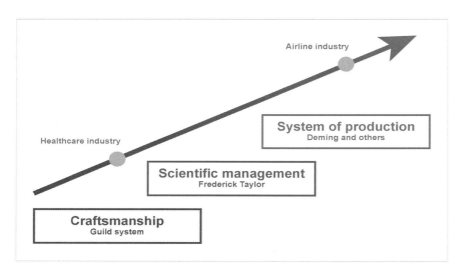

Figure 18: Evolution of process management

among doctors. And most hospitals are still organized in a top-down fashion that is characteristic of Taylorism.

In contrast, the airline industry has moved toward a system of production. It uses very standardized, routine procedures and safety checks. Pilots go through highly rigorous, systematic training, including years of flight simulations. Because processes are highly standardized, each pilot receives the same information during training and while in the air.

The application of modern improvement methods to healthcare

The improvement methods promoted by Deming, Womack and others are highly applicable in the complex healthcare delivery environment. The Institute for Healthcare Improvement (IHI) has published many papers and other documents demonstrating how to use these modern-day improvement techniques in healthcare.

Although poor quality and waste are common in healthcare, quality improvement and Lean methods are not typically associated with care delivery. However, the principles of quality improvement and Lean management can work in healthcare as well as they work in other industries. These are strategies that can be applied to any organization that seeks to improve processes and eliminate waste.

Any organization — including a healthcare organization — achieves its outcomes through a series of interlinked processes that are intended to create value for its customers. This implies a clear understanding of who the customer really is. Because of healthcare's complexity and silos that exist within the system, it has not been uncommon to confuse internal customers — physicians, hospitals, payers, etc., — with the ultimate customers: patients. This is a distinction that healthcare providers must understand if they are going to successfully adapt to future demands for value-based outcomes that benefit patients, communities and society.

The goal of quality improvement and Lean methods is to distinguish value-added from non-value added steps in a process and to eliminate as many non-value added steps as possible while optimizing the value added steps. The ultimate goal for healthcare is to optimize value for patients. In order to maximize value, healthcare leaders and front-line clinicians must understand value in terms of what patients and communities need and want from the healthcare delivery system. They must then map every step of any given process — the so-called value stream —

> " In order to maximize value, healthcare leaders and front-line clinicians must understand value in terms of what patients and communities need and want from the healthcare delivery system. They must then map every step of any given process — the so-called value stream — and eliminate any step that does not produce value. "

and eliminate any step that does not produce value. Furthermore, they must optimize the remaining steps to maximize quality and efficiency. If this is done successfully, value will flow from beginning to end in a process based on pull (i.e., the expressed needs of patients).

When Lean principles are applied rigorously throughout an organization, they have been demonstrated to have a dramatic effect on quality, throughput, productivity, waste reduction and cost. In other industries, it is not uncommon for improvements to range up to 90 percent.[70]

A growing list of leading-edge organizations are demonstrating that these improvement techniques can be effective in improving the quality of care, reducing harm, improving patient satisfaction, reducing waste and lowering costs. Under the visionary leadership of Brent James, MD, David A. Burton, MD, and others, Utah-based Intermountain Healthcare has demonstrated two decades of success implementing improvement principles promoted by Deming, Womack and others to achieve superior outcomes in quality, safety, waste reduction and cost savings. Many of Intermountain Healthcare's achievements in the area of quality improvement (e.g., reduction of adverse drug events, lowering infection rates, eliminating unnecessary C-sections, improving ventilator management, etc.,) and their application of information technology and analytics to support data-driven improvement are phenomenal and deserve widespread emulation.

Similar results are being achieved by other leading-edge healthcare organizations. For example, the Virginia Mason Hospital and Medical Clinic (VMMC) in Seattle, Washington, began implementing Lean principles in 2002. Since the introduction of Lean, they have demonstrated they can save capital, use staff more efficiently, reduce inventories, improve productivity, save space and improve quality. Improvements have resulted in tens of millions of dollars in savings.

There are many additional facets to Lean thinking and its application to healthcare. Readers interested in delving deeper into Lean are encouraged to read the IHI white paper entitled "Going Lean in Healthcare."[71]

Eventually, all healthcare organizations, regardless of payer models, will need to emulate the efforts of these improvement pioneers if they want to survive the future transformation of healthcare. Given the increasing focus on value in healthcare, it can easily be argued that these techniques will be at the core of any healthcare delivery organization's ability to weather the coming changes.

Implications of modern improvement methods for clinicians

The success of these methods in clinical care delivery is not surprising to any experienced clinician who also understands these improvement strategies. After all, quality improvement in healthcare — as in any other industry — is simply the result of applying the science of process management. Although complex, healthcare delivery is basically a system made up of thousands of interlinked processes. A process can be defined as a series of linked steps, often but not necessarily sequential, that are designed to produce a specific outcome or set of outcomes resulting in value for patients. Process management implies that one starts with the right knowledge of processes, systems (processes interacting together), human psychology, good data and an understanding of variation. It further suggests that one builds a rational system to manage processes and ongoing learning.

It is worth noting that this approach will be empowering for clinicians, the front-line workers, or smart-cogs, of healthcare delivery. The core business of any healthcare organization is delivering clinical care. Value in healthcare implies the delivery of high-quality, safe, effective care, efficiently delivered with minimal waste and a high degree of compassion. Effectively managing clinical care implies one effectively manages the processes of care. It does not imply managing physicians and other clinicians. Only well-trained, conscientious clinicians can effectively manage the process of care.

Value in healthcare will be achieved only by engaging clinicians, the front-line workers of healthcare delivery, and supporting their ability to optimize workflow, standardize processes and reduce waste while also being able to reasonably adapt to individual patient needs. From a workforce perspective, healthcare is very fortunate. Few industries have a workforce that is as talented, well-educated and committed to serving the customer as does healthcare. The vast majority of clinicians get up every day with the desire to be the best they can be for the patients they serve. The goal of management is to provide them the training, tools, techniques, data, environment and other forms of support they need to be successful in the quest for value.

> " Effectively managing clinical care implies one effectively manages the processes of care. It does not imply managing physicians and other clinicians. Only well-trained, conscientious clinicians can effectively manage the process of care. "

Having said that, going down this road will also require that clinicians give up on the craft-based approach of medicine. The traditional craft-based approach to medicine has consisted of an individual physician putting the healthcare needs of an individual patient before any other end or goal and drawing on his or her clinical knowledge gained through education and experience to develop a unique diagnostic and treatment regimen that is customized for that individual patient. In the modern era, healthcare has simply become too complex and too costly to rely on this traditional approach to deliver the right care to the right patient at the right time, every time, while also assuring that the overall population benefits.

Few would argue that the healing professions are not changing. Care has simply become too complex not to go in a new direction. The profession of medicine is going through a fundamental shift from a traditional craft-based practice to a more sophisticated profession-based practice. Perhaps more accurately, this could be described as a multidisciplinary team-based method of practice. While it has always been true, medicine is now becoming even more a team-based endeavor.

> "The profession of medicine is going through a fundamental shift from a traditional craft-based practice to a more sophisticated profession-based practice. Perhaps more accurately, this could be described as a multidisciplinary team-based method of practice. While it has always been true, medicine is now becoming even more a team-based endeavor.

A profession-based practice consists of groups of clinical peers treating similar patients in a shared setting using carefully coordinated and standardized care delivery processes (i.e., evidence-based order sets, protocols) that individual clinicians can adapt based on specific patient characteristics or needs across the care pathways. It is noteworthy that this approach emulates the Lean concepts that include standardization, yet also allows for adapting to individual customer needs.

This new environment implies that clinicians are operating in a highly supportive and rational care delivery and improvement system that allows them to optimally manage care processes while collecting data to support continuous improvement and learning. Finally, there is growing evidence that this profession-based approach is less complex and less expensive and that it produces better outcomes for patients and communities. Such a system can also be an empowering and satisfying work environment for clinicians.

There are signs of this change everywhere. Most patients already have multiple physicians and dozens of other caregivers involved in their care. Integrated care delivery systems are being formed. Care delivery environments are increasingly supported by advanced information technology, including electronic health records (EHRs), decision support systems and analytic systems. Internists are now required to demonstrate knowledge of systems-based theory as part of the internal medicine certification process. These and other signs point to the fact that these trends are real, inevitable and lasting.

Clearly, the solo-based practice is dying. At the national medical association level, the awareness and acceptance of this shift has largely already occurred, but it is not happening as quickly at the individual physician level. It is time for all clinicians to consider this new, highly empowering approach to clinical care delivery.

Given the complexity of the field, healthcare organizations would benefit enormously from developing a systematic approach to improvement. It is useful to have a framework to discuss improvement, such as the Health Catalyst approach that uses three systems for effective care delivery, as illustrated in Figure 19: an analytic system, a deployment system and a content system. Achieving scalable and sustainable outcomes requires effectively implementing these three systems.

The first system, the analytic system (see Figure 20), is where an organization standardizes the way it measures things, including calculations and definitions. It's also where the enterprise data warehouse (EDW) and data visualizations reside.

To strengthen and improve analytic systems, organizations need to first unlock the data. This requires implementing a well-designed analytical infrastructure, automating information distribution, and the ability to identify patterns in the data. The Health Catalyst Late-Binding™ Data Warehouse platform, metadata engine and the Late Binding data bus represent one example of this type of analytical infrastructure. Using the Health Catalyst foundational applications and common visualization engine, healthcare organizations can successfully automate the distribution of information. They can also use the Health Catalyst discovery and advanced applications to discover patterns in data.

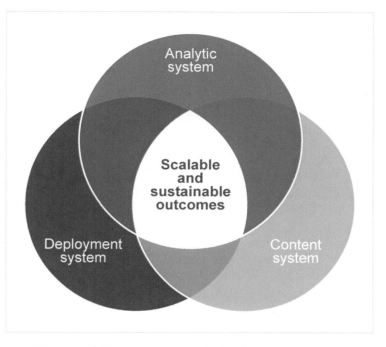

Figure 19: Three systems of effective care delivery

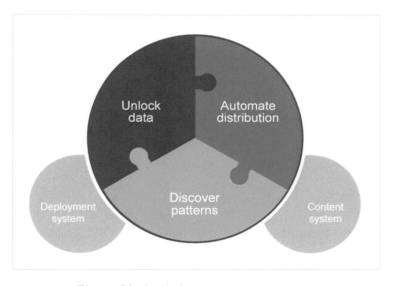

Figure 20: Analytic system components

The second system, the deployment system, illustrated in Figure 21, involves standardizing organizational work. To improve deployment systems, an organization needs to start by organizing permanent teams that take ownership of the quality, cost and patient satisfaction associated with care delivery. The organization also needs to organize team structures, provide training on roles, allow teams to design their own solutions and make

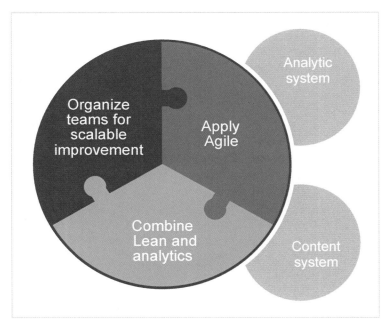

Figure 21: Deployment system components

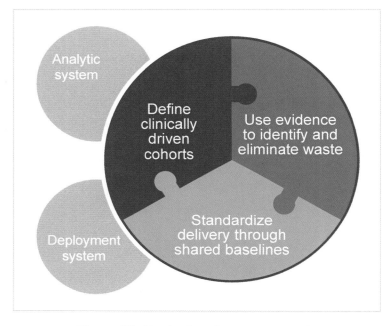

Figure 22: Content system components

sure improvements are implemented consistently. Encouraging physicians and nurses to design new ways of doing things creates a sense of ownership in the solution they come up with. This is called fingerprinting, and it is encouraged. An organization also needs to implement an agile, or iterative, method, which fosters continuous improvement. Organizations need to integrate Lean process improvement with measurement systems so they can have immediate, automated feedback on performance in addition to a historical view. All of these activities help organizations spread and sustain their improvement gains.

The third system, the content system, involves standardizing medical knowledge work (see Figure 22). Even when a new study comes out and identifies best practices, it can take as long as 17 to 20 years for physicians to integrate the new knowledge into everyday practices.[72] By standardizing knowledge assets, such as order sets, intervention criteria, value stream maps and patient safety protocols, an organization can improve the speed at which new medical knowledge becomes everyday practice. This process includes a consistent standard method for gathering evidence, evaluating that evidence, and integrating it into care delivery.

To help strengthen content systems, an organization needs to define their groups of patients (cohorts) and identify and eliminate various types of waste that occur when work is not standardized. Then, it needs to speed up the integration of evidence into everyday care delivery and standardize delivery of care by using shared baselines.

By leveraging all of the components of the analytic, deployment and content systems, an organization can truly ignite change in behavior throughout the entire care delivery system. And by igniting change through analytic, deployment and content systems, healthcare delivery organizations can achieve scalable and sustainable outcomes by unlocking data, assembling permanent teams focused on ongoing process improvement and creating knowledge assets that make the right thing to do the easy thing to do.

In the following chapters, we will discuss each of the three systems in more detail, reviewing the steps an organization needs to take to improve them, discussing the concepts an organization needs to understand to improve care and discovering what results it can expect from igniting change.

4 THE ANALYTICS SYSTEM: STANDARD MEASUREMENT WORK

An overview of the three-system framework for improving and sustaining clinical effectiveness, reducing waste and improving patient safety was discussed in chapter 3. Now we will review the analytic system.

This discussion will focus on unlocking your data and the importance of a good measurement system. By the end of this chapter, you should be able to describe different data models (including their strengths and weaknesses in healthcare), know how to use Pareto analysis to prioritize improvement opportunities, and discover patterns in the data to ignite meaningful, scalable and sustainable change.

Arguably, healthcare is the most data-intense industry in the world. Clinicians cannot deliver and sustain high-quality, safe care without information that is readily available. Measurement is the basis for assessing and sustaining potential improvements in healthcare quality. Deming once said, "In God we trust, all others must bring data." In order to know whether a change is an improvement, an analytic system is absolutely essential. Key performance measures allow improvement teams to assess care against past performance (shared common baselines), evidence-based clinical guidelines and nationally recognized standards. As Lord Kelvin said, "If you cannot measure it, you cannot improve it." In an improvement effort, you always need some form of objective measure to demonstrate how well things are working.

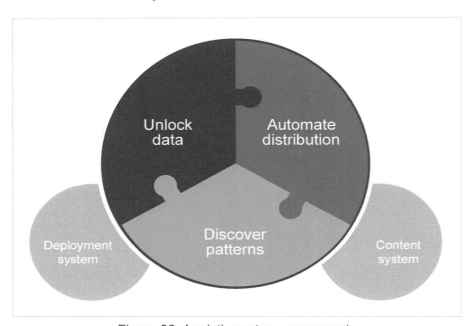

Figure 23: Analytic system components

Analytics have to do with how we make data accessible for use, how we use data, how we measure work, how we prioritize improvement opportunities and how we monitor improvement efforts over time. The three components of an analytic system are shown in Figure 23. First, an organization needs to effectively unlock their data. Second, an organization needs to broadly distribute the data to individuals across the organization and teach them how to access and use the data — so-called self-serve analytics, versus the current report-queue mentality where one requests and waits for a report to be built that may or may not meet their needs. And, third, improvement teams need to discover patterns in the data so they can target areas for improvement, and ignite meaningful and sustainable change. We'll discuss each of these components in turn, starting with unlocking data.

Two ways of using data: accountability versus learning

Few would argue that data is necessary to drive improvement. However, it is equally important to understand at the outset of an improvement initiative how data should be used to optimize the likelihood that clinicians will engage in improvement efforts.

New knowledge and a migration to a profession-based model of care require a move from the traditional judgment-based model to a learning-based model. A judgment-based approach focuses on the person, while a learning-based model focuses on continuous improvement.

A judgment-based approach tends to make most people defensive and creates resistance to learning. Therefore, it will likely impede continuous improvement. Based on the philosophy that the best defense is a good offense, the accused will often counterattack in an attempt to shift the blame elsewhere. In an attempt to kill the messenger, they may challenge the veracity of the accuser, the validity of the analytic system, the accuracy of the data, the legitimacy of the analytical methods and the accuracy of the evaluation. They will also often question the competence and motives of those conducting the assessment. This is a classic example of the cycle of fear described by Scherkenbach and illustrated in Figure 24.[73] The behaviors described in the cycle of fear occur because the majority of situations where errors occur are the result of a flawed system rather than a failure by an individual.

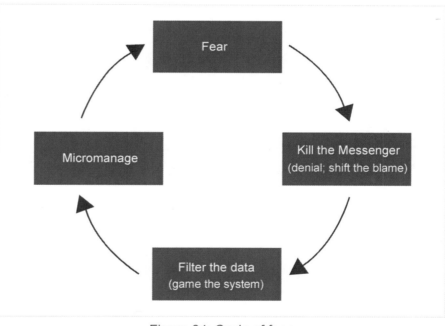

Figure 24: Cycle of fear

Brent James, MD, of Intermountain Healthcare, Don Berwick, MD — the founder of the Institute for Healthcare Improvement (IHI) and former administrator of the Centers for Medicare and Medicaid Services (CMS) — and Molly Coye, MD, chief innovation officer at UCLA, defined two ways of using data to get results.[74]

As illustrated in Figure 25, you can use data to hold people accountable or to measure improvement and encourage learning.

Every organization needs to gather some data that encourages accountability, but the overall focus should be on learning, not accountability or judgment.

The focus you choose will determine what you do to improve your numbers. Deming identified three ways to get a better number:

⊛ The first is to improve the system. To do this, you have to change your processes and add value at the front line.

⊛ The second is to suboptimize. You focus on improving the area being measured, often at the expense of other areas.

⊛ The third is to game the numbers. You manipulate the data to make the numbers look better. In healthcare, this is often accomplished by eliminating troublesome subpopulations from the cohort of patients.

A learning approach focuses on the process and the system. This is a bottoms-up approach centered on the idea that people can study a flawed process and improve it over time. A profession-based model allows and encourages people to continuously learn and improve. It involves them in the solution. Thus, a profession-based approach is essential to fostering a culture of continuous improvement in healthcare.

Organizations that focus on learning are more likely to improve their processes and systems. Organizations that focus on accountability are more likely to suboptimize or game the numbers.

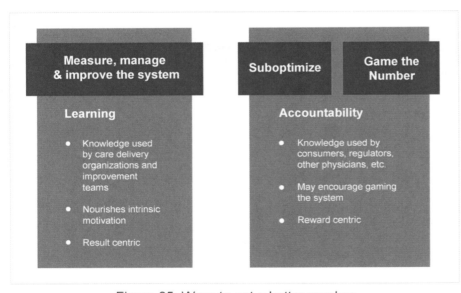

Figure 25: Ways to get a better number

What makes healthcare data unique?

There are several characteristics of healthcare data that make it unique. First of all, healthcare delivery and healthcare organizations are both diverse and complex. As a result, healthcare data tends to reside in multiple places and formats (e.g., text, numeric, paper, digital, pictures, videos, multimedia, etc.). Some healthcare data is structured, while other types of data are unstructured. Even in situations where clinicians should be putting data in a structured field, they may not be, resulting in the need to manually extract the data — a time-consuming and costly process. Oftentimes, healthcare data is described using inconsistent or variable definitions. For example, one group of clinicians may define a cohort of asthmatic patients differently than another group of clinicians. Healthcare also tends to generate very large volumes of data. The amount of new healthcare knowledge is massive and expanding on an almost daily basis. This means evidence is constantly changing. Regulatory and reporting requirements also continue to increase and evolve. Finally, for both care delivery and improvement efforts, clinicians need to get to patient-level detail.

The best way to make healthcare data accessible

A healthcare enterprise data warehouse (EDW) is the core of an analytical infrastructure. Given its complexity and quantity, it is important that healthcare data be readily accessible electronically and that the design of the EDW is maximally adaptable to support the dynamic and unique nature of the healthcare environment.

EDWs are described using conceptual data models. Different data models have been developed to meet various analytic requirements. A data model can be thought of as a diagram or flowchart that illustrates the relationships between data and data sources. The data model demonstrates the specific entities, attributes and relationships involved in a business or enterprise. The data model serves as the basis that IT professionals use to create the physical data model. The characteristics of the data model matter because of the complex and dynamic nature of healthcare data and the healthcare environment. Various types of data models and how they relate to healthcare are described below.

Data model types

There are several approaches to unlocking data in healthcare. One approach is the enterprise data model. In this model, an organization creates a perfect model of the data, representing all the concepts and relationships that need to be defined. They then map the different source transactional systems into that model, as shown in Figure 26.

This model works well in some industries — such as banking and retail — that have minimal variability in their

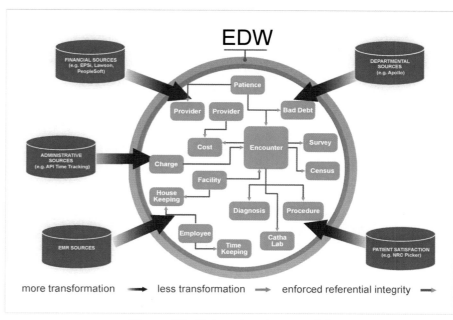

Figure 26: Enterprise data model
(View Appendix C for larger version)

data and where concepts and definitions are relatively static. Unfortunately, this highly organized model cannot be delivered incrementally, it takes a long time to create and it can be expensive. The extract, transform and load (ETL) routines used to move data into the model are complex. Finally, because of the characteristics of healthcare data — including constant, evidence-based care updates — you have to continuously redesign the model to make new data fit. Some healthcare systems have spent years on this approach and still have not been able to move any data into the model. This model has had limited success in healthcare, although it has been very successful in other industries.

Another approach to unlocking data is the dimensional data model, as illustrated in Figure 27. With this model, an organization builds an analytic data mart for a particular area — such as heart failure — gathers the data it needs directly from the source systems and maps it to different areas.

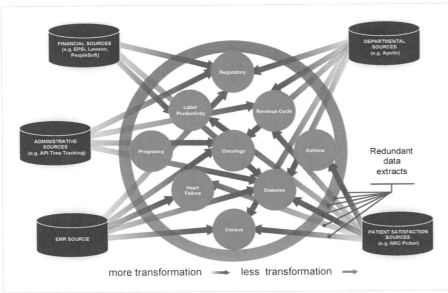

Figure 27: Dimensional data model
(View Appendix C for larger version)

This model is easy to start. However, it grows very quickly, as do the data streams, until several redundant streams exist. This creates a challenge for those trying to maintain the model. If one underlying source system changes, they have to change each extraction routine that uses that particular source. Additionally, it often doesn't have underlying patient-level detail. If a metric in a summary mart is unfavorable, you are unable to drill to the patient level to determine the reasons why.

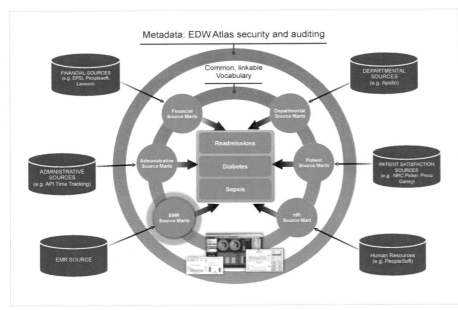

Figure 28: Late-Binding™ Data Warehouse
(View Appendix C for larger version)

A new approach to data modeling that Health Catalyst uses to address healthcare's unique data needs is the Late-Binding™ Data Warehouse (Figure 28). The advantages of the late binding approach are that it is generally faster to launch, it is easier and less expensive to maintain, and most importantly, it provides maximum adaptability for clinicians who are involved in improving care in the highly dynamic healthcare environment.

In the late binding model, one brings data into the warehouse in a raw format that keeps the same structure and feel of the underlying transactional system. This quick copy can be done in a few weeks, unlike the enterprise model, which can take years to develop. The structure stays the same, which enables analysts familiar with the transactional system to recognize the data structure in the warehouse. Naming and data type standards are applied to make it easier for analysis, but minimal transformation occurs.

In the late binding platform one can connect disparate data with a common linkable vocabulary. For example, identifiers for patients, providers and facilities can be linked across different data source systems such as an electronic health record (EHR) or claims (source marts), and one patient can be viewed across the entire system. From there, you can build marts focused on a particular clinical area such as diabetes (subject area marts). This can be done quickly because you are not going back to the individual source systems. You already have all the data in the late binding data warehouse. If an underlying source changes, you update one extraction routine instead of multiple streams. The result is just-in-time data binding. Rather than trying to define everything up front, you bind the data later, when you are trying to solve an actual clinical or operational problem. Finally, you can build graphical data visualizations atop the subject area marts, so it's easier to interpret the data and identify trends and patterns.

> "In the late binding model, one brings data into the warehouse in a raw format that keeps the same structure and feel of the underlying transactional system. This quick copy can be done in a few weeks, unlike the enterprise model, which can take years to develop."

Data binding and why it matters

Data binding is a technique in which raw data elements are mapped to conceptual definitions. One of the keys to the data model developed by Health Catalyst is binding the data late (i.e., when clinicians are trying to solve a problem). But that doesn't mean you always wait until the end. Data that is stable, like vocabulary terms and patient and provider identifiers, can be bound early. Data that is likely to change should be bound later. For example, length of stay (LOS) in a hospital may sound straightforward on paper, but surgeons might define LOS as point of incision to discharge from the post-anesthesia care unit (PACU), and cardiologists might define it as emergency department (ED) arrival to discharge. Because the LOS definition will change for different use cases, you will want to bind it later.

Figure 29 shows points where you can bind data.

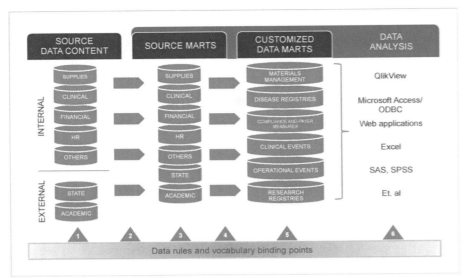

Figure 29: Early versus late binding
(View Appendix C for larger version)

> The earliest you can bind data is when you are moving it from transactional systems into the warehouse and then during the ETL process (points 1 and 2 in Figure 29). It is best to bind only low-volatile rules and vocabularies at these first points.

> You can also bind data in the target data source model they land in or when moving it to customized data marts (points 3 and 4).

> You can bind somewhat volatile data in the customized data mart — this is still considered late binding (point 5).

> The last place you can bind data is in the visualization layer for rules and vocabulary that are likely to change. Once you establish definitions, the data can be locked down (points 3, 4 or 5).

A late binding data warehouse has several advantages, including:

> The process is driven by business and clinical needs instead of architectural design.

> It is less expensive to develop because it can be built in stages.

> The late binding approach provides both atomic- and summary-level information, so you are not bombarded with data, yet you can find specifics when you need them.

> It is flexible and allows an organization to build other structures on top of it, if desired.

> It is very quick and easy to develop and deploy source and subject area data marts, so an organization can start using and benefiting from it sooner.

> It becomes a great source of analytic information for different departments.

- The structure aligns with governance or data stewardship, so different departments can access different source marts because they are the stewards of that data.

- It improves an organization's information about the data (i.e., metadata) by tracking how often it is refreshed, where it came from, who's in charge of that data and so on.

It is noteworthy that the late binding data warehouse is the approach that has most consistently worked in healthcare to unlock data and drive improved results.

Automating data distribution

Once the data is unlocked, an organization can automate the broad distribution of the information. Ideally, the data is distributed electronically to enable clinicians to effectively and efficiently view the information they need in as close to real time as possible.

Today, in most healthcare delivery organizations, the distribution work falls primarily to analysts or clinicians, who encounter many challenges. First, they must understand what types of data are needed. Before they can locate and compile that data, they have to wait for IT to run reports or queries. Only then can they start interpreting data and distributing it to the right people. Obviously, understanding the need and interpreting data are two value-add tasks. But at many healthcare organizations at least 80 percent of the analyst's or clinician's time is spent gathering or waiting for data instead of analyzing information.

There are several examples of non-value-added tasks. If the person preparing the report doesn't get all the necessary data, he or she has to do chart abstraction, where one pulls up the patient's record and manually types the missing data into an Excel spreadsheet or another data collection file system. This is sometimes called sneaker ETL because the analyst spends a lot of time walking from one system to another to enter data. When you reach the stage where you want to provide others access to the data (i.e., the distribution/provisioning stage), the new data are typically integrated into another Excel spreadsheet (spreadsheet data marts or spreadmarts), but they aren't tied back to the source information. The person creating the report might have built clever macros to grab this data, but if they leave the organization, they also take the knowledge about how the macros work, and the people left behind can only hope the data imports correctly. Spreadmarts are volatile — they are not standardized, they are not predictable and they are often not secure.

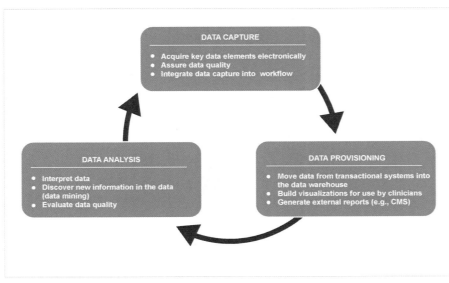

Figure 30: Automating data gathering

Automation can help solve these problems, as illustrated in Figure 30. An organization can easily eliminate unused or obsolete reports and standardize data capture as part of the workflow during or just after key events. Instead of sending reports, an organization can encourage front-line workers to explore data themselves by collecting data in the EDW, standardizing common definitions and automating information distribution. Finally, an organization can use rollup instead of summary data by gathering patient-level detail and using it as a starting point for summaries. This allows end-users to drill down and answer "why" questions that might otherwise go unanswered.

By automating data capture, data distribution (provisioning) and data analysis, an organization can encourage self-exploration. It is best if healthcare can get away from a report factory mentality where an end-user sends in a data request and waits a couple of weeks or longer for the results. If an end-user wants the request moved up the list, they need to cajole the IT person to do them a favor — and hope the data is right when they get it back. Often, the end-user has forgotten the question they originally asked because it takes so long to get the report. By getting rid of this report factory mentality, and making tools that the end-user can use available, the end-user can explore their own data and ask and answer their own questions.

Some organizations feel as though they have automated their data because they have created dashboards. When mandated from the top, dashboards can create fire drills that steal clinicians' time and attention. They often do not match the front-line clinical needs or workflow and overemphasize a single outcome metric while neglecting far more important process metrics. Executives do need information, but ideally, problems should be attacked at the clinical level, using metrics designed at the frontline. Rather than a one-off request for a single outcome metric, the executive team may want to track a department's progress toward achieving a set of core objectives that have been defined by the department to help improve outcomes.

Chapter 4.2 — Prioritizing improvement opportunities

Once an organization's data is unlocked and readily available, the next step in the improvement journey is to decide where to focus improvement efforts. Every organization has limited resources. Their goal is to get the greatest benefit from the resources they invest in improvement efforts. Therefore, they need to determine which investments will provide the greatest benefit: improving care for the largest number of patients, streamlining operations to the greatest extent possible and lowering costs. Taking this approach will help organizations achieve their highest value.

The Anatomy of Healthcare Delivery — a conceptual framework for organizing healthcare

Anyone involved in healthcare delivery knows it is complex. Traditionally, healthcare has used clinical service lines to categorize clinical care. While clinical service lines may be useful, they are generally not comprehensive enough to capture all clinical care. A clinical service line model tends to be acute care-centric, and it does not adequately describe the details of any given care delivery process (e.g., what the decision points are, how decisions are made or who makes them). In short, the traditional clinical service line model does not provide us with the level of detail and the depth of understanding necessary to organize our thinking and manage the process of care most effectively. Thus, the need for a conceptual framework that supports our ability to do this.

This section focuses on a framework that lays out the process of healthcare delivery and provides context for a discussion about quality improvement opportunities. The framework accounts for population-based improvements in utilization as well as improvements in prevention, encounters or cases.

As healthcare increasingly focuses on producing value — higher quality and safer care at the lowest possible cost — there will be a shift in emphasis toward managing care across the continuum. There will be a need to efficiently and effectively conceptualize and manage care from the home to the clinic, urgent care unit, emergency department, special procedure unit or hospital.

As the pressure grows to manage care more effectively, there will be an increasing emphasis on post-acute care in order to reduce hospital lengths of stay or bypass the acute care admission altogether. Examples of post-acute care environments may include the home, clinic, home healthcare, skilled nursing facilities and hospice, as shown in Figure 31.

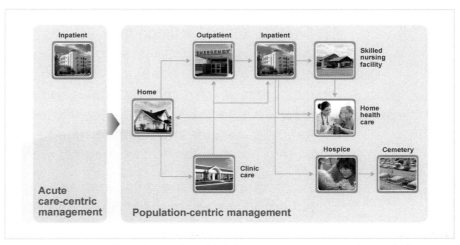

Figure 31: Population Health Management — paradigm shift

As healthcare transformation unfolds, a paradigm shift is taking place from an acute care-centric model of patient care to a focus on the continuum of care and a shift toward population-centric management. Some of this is being driven by federal government programs such as the Patient Protection and Affordable Care Act or the commercial emulation of value-based reimbursement in various forms that promote shared accountability for the risk and the reward of taking care of patients.

Conceptualizing the flow of care

The first step in understanding clinical care is to understand the flow of care when patients interact with the delivery system. The Anatomy of Healthcare Delivery framework developed by David A. Burton, MD, and shown in Figure 32, demonstrates the potential pathways patients can go through in their interactions with the delivery system. This is a conceptual framework that enables us to organize our thinking about the care delivery process and to focus our attention on key processes and decision-making points. The degree to which an organization standardizes their approach in each of the knowledge asset categories (indicated by the blue and light blue boxes shown in Figure 32) will impact the degree of variation in care delivery.

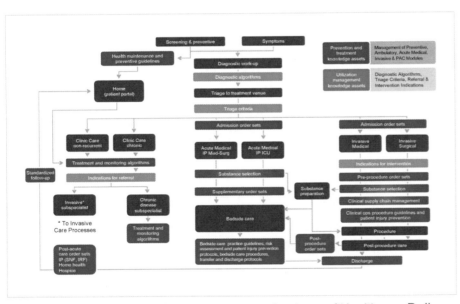

Figure 32: Population health management — Anatomy of Healthcare Delivery
(View Appendix C for larger version)

As seen at the top of Figure 32, patients may present with symptoms or they may be seeking screening or preventive care. If they have symptoms, or there are positive findings identified in the process of screening, patients enter into a diagnostic workup. Once a provisional diagnosis is established, patients are triaged to a treatment venue (e.g., clinic, acute medical or invasive) based on decisions that are driven more by subjective considerations than objective data. The goal should be to triage the patient to the care venue that best matches delivery system resources to the patient's needs in a manner that optimizes the balance between quality, safety and cost (e.g., ambulatory, acute medical or invasive).

Condition-specific care guidelines and implementation protocols can be developed for each of the boxes in the flow of care. Health maintenance and preventive guidelines are applied to patients who neither have symptoms of disease nor show positive results after screening. These guidelines, which extend to the patient's home, help keep those who are healthy in a state of good health for as long as possible.

Knowledge assets focused on the care processes are employed in the management of preventive, ambulatory, acute medical, invasive and post-acute care. Treatment and monitoring algorithms are used to care for patients in ambulatory clinics. If they have a positive diagnosis, a sequence of events is launched. For example, treatment of a diabetic usually starts with diet and exercise. If these initial efforts do not achieve treatment goals, the next step is to prescribe a single oral agent for type 2 diabetes, followed by addition of a second oral agent if treatment goals are not reached, and so on down to basic insulin therapy if oral agents do not work.

If after a defined period of time treatment such as that outlined above for type 2 diabetes fails to meet the established aim, the patient may be referred to a chronic disease subspecialty clinic where more intensive treatment algorithms are employed.

Some patients for whom adequate care is not possible in a clinic environment, or who are sick enough to be triaged directly to the acute medical or invasive venues of care, receive care in one of these acute care venues. These types of patients are triaged to specific care units within these venues based on their condition and acuity. Admission order sets for these patients regulate their care during the initial phase of their treatment.

As treatment progresses on an acute medical unit, supplementary orders govern care in accordance with evidence-based guidelines for administration of blood products, pharmaceuticals or fluid and electrolyte replacement.

For the invasive care units, there are pre-procedure order sets that include clinical supply chain management processes such as the utilization of prosthetic devices (e.g., hip or knee replacement), stents, synthetic grafts, devices to regulate heart rhythm or neurostimulators.

For patients admitted directly to acute medical care units, the various order sets translate into bedside care practice guidelines, including risk assessments and intervention protocols to prevent patient injury, protocols designed to deliver standard evidence-based care for the patient's condition, and ultimately transfer and discharge protocols. Similarly, for patients who undergo treatment in invasive care units, there are care practice guidelines such as "timeouts" and sponge and instrument counts to prevent wrong site surgeries and retained foreign bodies. After a procedure is completed in one of the invasive care units, post-anesthesia care is initiated, based on post-procedure order sets.

As the patient enters post-acute care, there are order sets for facilities such as skilled nursing facilities, inpatient rehabilitation facilities, home health and hospice, as well as standardized follow-up instructions as the patient eventually returns home. Standardized steps and treatments are employed in each venue of care.

In addition to the treatment cascades outlined above, which apply within an episode or case of care, there are complementary criteria or algorithms that determine what tests should be ordered based on diagnostic findings, as shown in Figure 32. For example, once a provisional diagnosis is established, specific triage criteria are used. An example of this is the CURB-65 criteria for community-acquired pneumonia. Documenting how many of the risk factors are present helps the clinician decide whether it is safe to treat in the ambulatory environment or whether the patient needs to be admitted to a med-surg general acute care unit or to an intensive care unit.

In the clinic care setting, the treatment and monitoring algorithms lead to indications for referral if the care process does not achieve established goals and target values. For example, a diabetic who is treated in accordance with the standardized steps of the algorithm but does not achieve the target hemoglobin A1c level within a defined time window meets indications for referral to an endocrinologist. Another example of indications for referral would be a child with acute otitis media that, after recurrent infections, progresses into serous otitis media, with complicating speech retardation and/or hearing loss. Such a child needs to be referred to an ear, nose and throat (ENT) specialist for evaluation and possible myringotomy and placement of tympanostomy tubes.

Similarly, patients who are referred to an invasive physician (i.e., interventional medical or surgical subspecialist) either during the acute phase of their illness or after failing to respond appropriately to clinic care treatment and monitoring algorithms, should also meet indications for intervention before an invasive procedure is undertaken.

A Clinical Integration hierarchy — care process families and clinical programs

Now that we have examined how patients flow through the care delivery system and its critical decision points, we can use the information to create a logical framework to help us organize a Clinical Integration hierarchy to help us think about clinical care delivery. This hierarchy applies along the continuum of care delivery, from the home and clinic, to the outpatient and inpatients venues of acute care, and thence to the post-acute care venues.

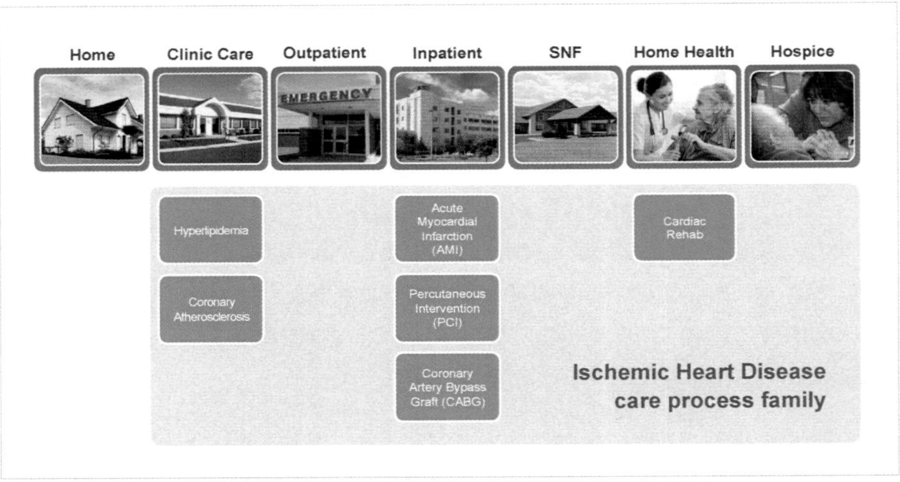

The most granular level of the hierarchy is the care process. Figure 33 shows examples of ischemic heart disease care processes (e.g., hyperlipidemia, coronary atherosclerosis, AMI, PCI, CABG and cardiac

Figure 33: Clinical Integration hierarchy — care process families
(View Appendix C for larger version)

rehab). These care processes belong to the next level of the hierarchy, the ischemic heart disease care process family.

Ischemic heart disease and its care process family siblings of heart failure, heart rhythm disorders and vascular disorders make up the cardiovascular clinical program, which is an example of the next level of the hierarchy. These care process families make up the vast majority of clinical conditions in the cardiovascular domain, as illustrated in Figure 34.

The cardiovascular clinical program is one of several major clinical domains, as shown in Figure 35. Clinical programs are organized based on physician specialists and other clinicians who share management of care processes and who are responsible for the ordering of care for patients. Either they work on things together, or one team's output is another team's input (e.g., OB-GYN subspecialists and neonatologists). Each of these domains or clinical programs consists of a group of care process families.

Clinical support services deliver care ordered by clinical program physicians

Once care is ordered by clinical program physicians, clinical support services are responsible for delivering care to patients. Clinical support services, as illustrated in Figure 36, include diagnostic,

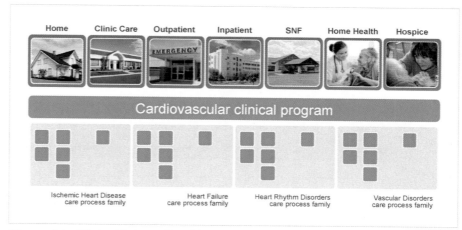

Figure 34: Clinical Integration hierarchy — cardiovascular clinical program
(View Appendix C for larger version)

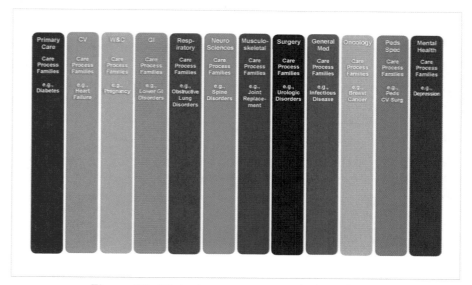

Figure 35: Clinical programs — ordering of care
(View Appendix C for larger version)

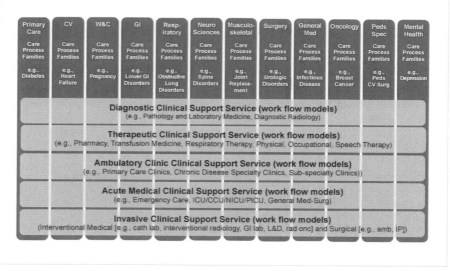

Figure 36: Clinical support services — delivery of care
(View Appendix C for larger version)

therapeutic, clinic care, acute medical and invasive clinical support services. The vertical clinical programs order the care and are responsible for defining the evidence-based, scientific flow of the care. The horizontal clinical support services implement the care that is ordered and are responsible for defining a safe and efficient workflow.

Value Stream Map	Diagnostic CSS			Ambulatory CSS		Acute Medical CSS			Invasive CSS		
	Clin Path	Anat Path	Radi-ology	Peds	Adult	ECU	ICU/CCU	Med-Surg	IP Surg	ASC	Interv Med
Substances											
Pharmacy				X	X	X	X	X	X	X	X
Medications			X	X	X	X	X	X	X	X	X
Fluids						X	X	X	X	X	X
Electrolytes				X	X	X	X	X	X	X	X
Parenteral nutrition (TPN)						X	X	X	X		
Transfusion Medicine						X	X	X			
Glycemic Control (Glucose Mgmt)							X	X	X	X	
Healthcare Associated Infections											
Ventilator Associated Pneumonia							X				
Urinary Catheter Infections						X	X	X	X	X	X
Surgical Site Infections									X	X	X
Central Line Assoc Bldstream Inf						X	X	X	X		
Venous Thromboembolism							X	X	X	X	
Pressure Injury (Decubitus Ulcers)							X	X			
Falls (Strength, Agility, Cognition)						X	X	X			
Patient/Procedure Control									X	X	

Figure 37: Value stream protocols to help prevent patient injuries
(View Appendix C for larger version)

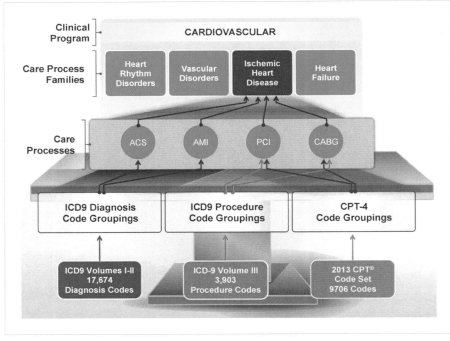

Figure 38: Mapping clinical programs to administrative codes

Patient injury prevention is an integral element of the workflow because patient injury really should be viewed as a defect in the implementation of optimal care. Figure 37 shows which value stream protocols each department should use to help prevent patient injuries.

In order to prioritize improvement projects relating to the ordering of care and its implementation, we need to be able to measure the relative size and variability of the three levels of the Clinical Integration hierarchy. This requires linking each level of the hierarchy to some quantitative metric, such as cost. This is done by mapping the clinical processes of care to administrative codes such as ICD-9-CM, diagnostic and procedure codes such as CPT-4 codes, and APR-DRGs. Figure 38 is a conceptual diagram that illustrates the use of a cardiovascular example using ICD-9-CM and CPT-4 codes. The ICD-9-CM codes are being supplanted by ICD-10-CM codes. ICD-10 will offer even more advantages because it can explain clinical conditions in far greater detail.

Medicare recently published nationwide data for the benefit of those developing innovation proposals. Using these data, one can group care by venue. Figure 39 illustrates the nationwide dollars of care based on venue: clinic care, outpatient, inpatient, skilled nursing facility, inpatient rehabilitation facility and home health and hospice. This helps us understand the relative contribution of each of the venues of care to the total Medicare expenditures nationwide.

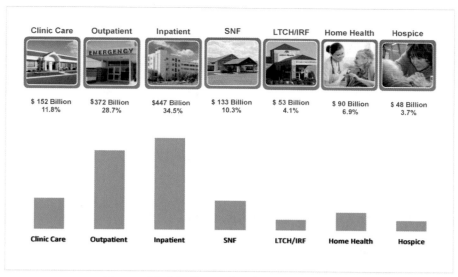

Figure 39: Medicare fee for service (FFS) payments by venue — 2008-2012

Key Process Analysis (KPA) — prioritizing the opportunity for variation improvement

The Anatomy of Healthcare Delivery framework helps clinicians and others understand the flow of patient care. It also provides a useful model for organizing the complex care delivery process and determining where to focus care improvement resources to achieve the greatest possible impact in terms of value. We will now turn our attention to a discussion of how we can use the Anatomy of Healthcare Delivery framework to prioritize improvement efforts.

The key variables in prioritization are resource consumption (larger processes offer greater opportunity) and variability. Once care process families are mapped to costs, relative resource consumption can be identified and ranked, as shown in Figure 40.

Each of the blue dots represents one of those care process families, such as arthritis, pregnancy, lower gastrointestinal disorders and so on. The red dots represent

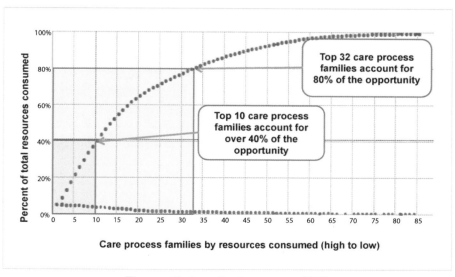

Figure 40: Inpatient per case KPA

the cumulative total of the blue dots. If you focus on the first 10 blue dots, the cumulative total is over 40 percent. This analysis looks at direct variable costs because they represent the costs over which providers have the most control.

Extending out to 32 processes, we reach a point of about 80 percent of total resource consumption. In addition to highlighting costs, this approach provides a reasonably good surrogate for the risk to the patient. For example, the higher the resource consumption, the more likely the patient is in an intensive and costly care environment such as the ICU. Both because of patient benefit and cost reduction opportunities, it is reasonable to assume that focusing on these 32 processes would yield the greatest benefit. Organizations would likely not be wise to invest money into processes on the far right of the grid because the benefit is less likely to outweigh the costs. If an organization is doing this, it may be prudent to refocus their improvement efforts on high-priority areas that offer a potentially greater return on investment.

One of the challenges that can be encountered when applying quality measures to different care process families is that many things cannot be compared, and hospitals lack clinical data that can be used to prioritize their problems. Instead of using clinical data they do not have, healthcare organizations can substitute financial data. This works surprisingly well because complicated, expensive care often entails greater risk to the patient. Additionally, financial variation often reveals clinical variation.

If the cost of care for the same type of patient varies greatly between two physicians at the same facility, the physicians are probably using different clinical practices. By standardizing on evidence-based practice, clinicians can improve outcomes and reduce costs. Financial data can be used to prioritize clinical initiatives, but it should not be used to confront physicians about cost. Improvement in cost outcomes should be a by-product of the standardization and improvement of clinical practices and not an end in itself.

Care process family	Case count rank	LOS hours (capacity) rank	Total charges rank	Total direct cost rank	Total direct cost opportunity rank	Organizational readiness (1 to 10) 1 = most ready
Trauma	9	2	2	3	3	7
Ischemic Heart Disease	3	7	1	2	2	3
Infectious Disease	6	3	3	1	1	6
Pregnancy	1	1	7	4	8	1
Heart Failure	10	8	4	5	5	5
Joints	11	13	8	6	16	9
Normal Newborn	2	6	20	24	32	2
GI Disorders	4	4	6	7	4	8
Lower Respiratory	5	5	5	8	6	4

Figure 41: Prioritization criteria and ranking

To prioritize the allocation of development resources, you want to combine and rank objective data criteria and subjective criteria, such as organizational readiness. Then, assess different care process families against those criteria as shown in Figure 41.

Pregnancy ranks first in case count and total LOS hours in Figure 41. Each delivery LOS is relatively short, but the number of deliveries makes pregnancy the top bed occupier. Pregnancy is only seventh in total charges because, on average, a labor and delivery event costs much less than a trauma or heart failure event. Infectious disease has the greatest variation in cost, which makes it an area of high opportunity as well.

We have gotten to a point where the data is readily accessible, and we have established a logical way to focus our efforts on the greatest areas of opportunity to maximize the return on our investments in quality improvement. The next step is to start identifying patterns in the data with the goal of measuring and sustaining improvements in care. Patterns in the data are often driven by variations. These include variations in clinician performance, data capture, data collection, processes, resource consumption and outcomes.

Before we discuss patterns in the data, it is important to touch on two important topics. First, we need to understand variations: types of variation, which variations matter and which do not, how we measure variation and how we monitor variation over time. As a part of this discussion we will review statistical process control (SPC), the most important quality improvement tool for identifying and monitoring variation. Second, we need to understand how to use data in quality improvement to maximize clinician engagement and outcomes. We will discuss each of these in turn and then go on to patterns in the data that help guide improvement efforts.

Understanding variation in healthcare

We live in the information age, and much of the information that bombards us every day comes in the form of numbers. In order to effectively use numerical information in decision making, however, we must be able to analyze, interpret and assimilate it. Unfortunately, few of us are taught how to make sense of numerical data. This is even true in the high-powered education that most clinicians receive. Arguably, clinicians work in the most information-intense industry in the world, yet they generally have not been taught the basics of analyzing and interpreting the volumes of data they encounter on a daily basis.

To understand information, it is important to grasp the concept of variation. Variation has been defined as a deviation from the norm, like the variation of colors in nature. A variation from an accepted standard can be important. For example, a variation in an electrocardiogram (EKG) tracing can tell a provider that a heart attack might be imminent. Not all variation is bad, of course. There are wide variations in people's appearance, for example. But these trait differences make each person unique.

> "We live in the information age, and much of the information that bombards us every day comes in the form of numbers. In order to effectively use numerical information in decision making, however, we must be able to analyze, interpret and assimilate it."

It is important to understand that variation exists in virtually all processes we encounter in work and in our daily lives. For example, people vary in looks, intelligence, how they learn, how they perform tasks, how they respond to events and how they perceive quality. In addition, the response of any given individual to a situation or process can vary over time.

Organizations are collections of people, and organizations can likewise vary as they respond to situations. Financial outcomes vary from company to company in the same industry and from quarter to quarter in the same company. Success rates for the same clinical procedure vary from physician group to physician group and from hospital to hospital. In addition, success rates for the same clinical procedure can vary for an individual physician group or hospital over time.

Clinicians constantly make decisions based on their interpretation of variations in information they encounter as they care for patients. Is it time for a patient to have a thorough clinical workup? Is a patient's condition improving, or should an alternative treatment be considered? Are the outcomes of the diabetics in my panel improving based on the treatment plan? Are we saving lives?

> The decisions we make are often based on whether we think the variation we observe is indicative of a true change or simply a random variation. Making this distinction between random variation and assignable cause variation (i.e., variation due to an identifiable cause instead of random events) is critically important in patient care. It is not possible to be a good clinician without knowing the difference.

The decisions we make are often based on whether we think the variation we observe is indicative of a true change or simply a random variation. Making this distinction between random variation and assignable cause variation (i.e., variation due to an identifiable cause instead of random events) is critically important in patient care. It is not possible to be a good clinician without knowing the difference.

There are numerous examples of how clinicians interpret patterns in variation as they practice clinical care every day. For three months in a row, the HgbA1c values in our panel of diabetic patients are higher than expected. Do the data indicate a trend that requires a change in how we are managing diabetes? What action should we take? A physician experiences some unexpected outcomes. As the chair of the clinical department, are these outcomes random variations, or should we intervene? Who needs special assistance and who should be left alone? The number of adverse events in a hospital is higher than last year's average for two months in a row. Should we respond with special programs, or is this simply a chance event?

It is important for clinicians to understand some of the basic concepts needed to accurately interpret variation. They must be able to determine whether the patterns of variation that are observed are indicative of a trend or simply a random variation similar to others observed in the past. Recognizing this distinction is essential to minimizing losses that can result from misinterpreting a pattern. These losses can include blaming people for problems that are beyond their control, spending money on interventions that are not necessary, wasting time looking for explanations of trends that do not matter and taking actions when it would have been better to do nothing.

Understanding systems and processes

In order to understand variation, it is helpful to appreciate the concepts of processes and systems. In his study of process in the 1920s, Walter Shewhart defined a process as a set of linked steps, often but not necessarily sequential, that are designed to cause some set of outcomes to occur, to transform inputs into outputs, to generate useful information and to add value.[75] Inputs to a process can include supplies, information or people. Outcomes from a process can include services, products or people.

A system has been defined as "an independent group of items, people or processes with a common purpose."[76] In this context, healthcare can be viewed as a complex system comprising thousands of interrelated processes.

Performance indicators for any process or system can be identified and measured. These performance indicators are referred to as quality characteristics. In clinical care, quality characteristics include rates of harm (e.g., adverse drug events, falls, retained foreign bodies, wrong site surgery, hospital acquired infections, handoff errors, etc.) and outcome measures (i.e., clinical outcomes, functional outcomes, satisfaction rates, access to care, rates of waste and cost outcomes).

> Performance indicators for any process or system can be identified and measured. These performance indicators are referred to as quality characteristics.

Quality characteristics will vary over time or by location. Analysis of variation in quality characteristics is used as a basis for taking action on the process or system. Deciding whether to act on variations in data depends on differentiating between variations that are inherently part of the process or system (so-called random or common cause variation) and those that are not part of the process or system (so-called assignable — or special cause — variation).

The output of a process can be graphed as a frequency distribution. A frequency distribution is a graphical representation of values of one or more variables sampled from a process, as seen in Figure 42. A frequency distribution tracks the performance of a process

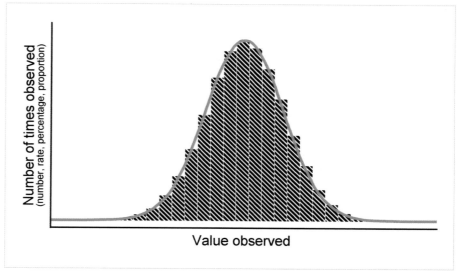

Figure 42: A frequency distribution

across a group of observations or measurements. It shows the number of times (y-axis — count, rate, proportion) each possible value occurred (x-axis). While it is not possible to exactly predict any single future observation for the process, the frequency distribution gives a range within which nearly all of the process's future measures are likely to fall. Stated another way, how a process behaved in the past is a reasonable predictor of how it will behave in the future.

Process capability is defined as the degree to which a process meets specifications. A specification explicitly states an acceptable range for a measurable performance or outcome parameter. This is usually expressed as the proportion of all measured points that fall within a specification range. A defect is a process output that does not meet specifications (i.e., an output that falls outside of the specification range).

The specification range is generally defined by control limits. Control limits represent action or decision thresholds. They generally are measured in units of standard deviations and are often referred to by the term "sigma scores." Six Sigma represents about 3 to 4 defects per million (six standard deviations from the mean). Five Sigma is about 5 to 6 defects per 100,000 (five standard deviations from the mean). Four Sigma is about 3 to 4 defects per 10,000 (four standard deviations from the mean). Three Sigma is about 4 to 5 defects per 1,000 (three standard deviations from the mean). Two Sigma is 4 to 5 defects per 100 (two standard deviations from the mean). One Sigma is about 30 to 40 defects per 100 (one standard deviation from the mean). Over time, you can build a graph of how often a process results in an output (outcome) that falls within specifications. Given this, you can measure the defect rate. This tells you how well a process works.

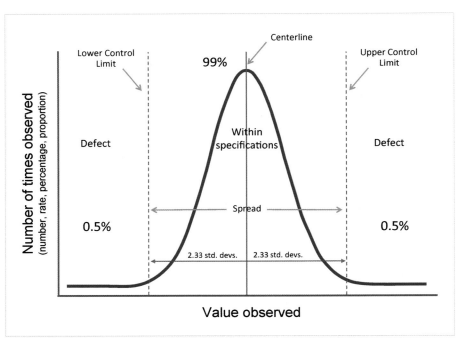

Figure 43: Frequency distribution within control limits

In frequency distributions, the parameters that drive the specification limits are the centerline and the spread. The centerline is the horizontal line on a control chart that represents the average for a process. The spread is bounded by the control limits for the process. These parameters explain how the random component of a process behaved in the past.

Figure 43 demonstrates a frequency distribution with the control limits set at 2.33 standard deviations from the mean such that 99 percent of the measurements are deemed acceptable and 1 percent of the measurements are deemed to be outside of specifications — that is, a 1 percent defect rate (0.5 percent of the defects below specifications and 0.5 percent of the defects above specifications).

Condition	Acceptable INR range
DVT/Pulmonary Embolus	2.0-3.0
Atrial Fibrillation	2.0-3.0
Anterior Myocardial Infarction (AMI)	2.5-3.5
Valve Replacement	2.5-3.5

Figure 44: Ideal range of coagulation for avoiding complications

Specification ranges are commonly used in healthcare. For example, specification ranges are often set based on a balance between an appropriate therapeutic range to avoid a clinical consequence and the need to minimize complications from the treatment. Coumadin anticoagulation is an example of this. Figure 44 demonstrates the range of coagulation that has been determined to be ideal for avoiding the most common complications of blood clots while also minimizing the risk of bleeding.

For any given population of patients on Coumadin, one can plot their Coumadin values in a frequency distribution. If the control limits are drawn narrowly, more patients will fall outside the ideal therapeutic range and risk the consequence of clots. If the control limits are defined over a broader range, more patients will avoid the risk of clots, but they will also face a higher risk of bleeding. For this reason, the majority of control limits in healthcare are drawn at three standard deviations from the mean (Three Sigma).

SPC and SPC control charts

A picture is worth a thousand words. This is a fundamental concept for quality improvement experts. Research has shown that the human eye can interpret patterns in graphical displays of data far better than in tables of numbers.[77-80] Rather than relying on confusing data tables, it is best to make a picture of the data and let the picture do the talking.

Plotting data over time offers insights and maximizes the learning from any data collected by revealing patterns and improvement opportunities. In quality improvement, SPC and SPC charts are key tools for providing pictures of data that can allow decision-makers to quickly determine whether variations are a likely or unlikely part of a process. If they are deemed to be unlikely, intervention may be necessary.

Shewhart, the physicist and statistician credited with initially pioneering SPC in managing processes, was initially presented with the challenge of improving and maintaining quality in the manufacture of telephone components. His approach to statistics was fundamentally different from many of his contemporaries. He adopted a strong operational focus, placing particular emphasis on understanding, measuring and improving processes. This led him to focus on using statistical methods that would allow him to better understand, analyze and measure variation in a process.

Shewhart studied Taylor-style mass production to better understand how processes worked. He recognized that the world we live in tends to follow physical laws. He also saw that complex processes tended to result in variable outputs. Shewhart then turned his attention to developing a deeper understanding of variation. Where did variation come from? What caused it?

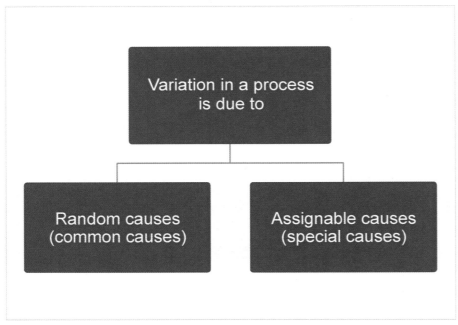

Figure 45: Sources of variation

Shewhart recognized that sources of variation at any point in a process can be one of two types: common (normal or chance) sources of variation and assignable sources of variation, as seen in Figure 45.

Most complex processes have many sources of variation. Most of these sources are minor and can be ignored. Such random variation represents the sum of many small variations arising from real, yet small causes that are inherent in any complex process or system. Random variation tends to follow the laws of probability. That is, it behaves as a statistically random function. Because random variation represents the sum of many small causes, it cannot be traced back to a root cause. Instead, it is a physical attribute of the process. It represents appropriate variation. Different processes have different levels of random variation. While random variation is an important part of measuring and monitoring a process, it is not useful in setting improvement goals for a process.

Because random variation is a physical attribute of a process, Shewhart recognized that the only way one can reduce random variation is to identify a new process that yields a better outcome and a new level of random variation. That is, a process that is superior to the original process. Managing random variation in this manner requires the use of the plan, do, study, act (PDSA) cycle.

The other type of variation Shewhart observed was special cause variation (later called "assignable variation" by Deming). Assignable variation represents variation that arises from a single cause that is not attributable to the process. Therefore, assignable variation can be identified, traced to a root cause and eliminated (or implemented if it improves the outcome of the process). Unwanted assignable variation represents inappropriate variation.

Identifying these two types of variation is important in quality improvement. If the dominant (assignable) sources of variation are identified, improvement teams can focus their attention on them. Improvement teams can track the assignable variation to its root cause. Once the root causes of the assignable variation sources are known, the team can eliminate them if they are found to contribute to less than optimal outcomes. Once an assignable cause of variation is removed, the process is said to be stable. Alternatively, if an assignable cause of variation represents an improvement, improvement teams can retain and exploit it in a new, stable process. When a process is stable, its variation should remain within a known set of limits. This stability will persist until another assignable source of variation is introduced.

Shewhart pioneered the use of SPC in managing and controlling processes and developed the control chart as a tool to use in differentiating random variation from assignable variation. SPC uses statistical methods to observe the performance of a process in order to predict significant variations that may result in a substandard outcome.

Creating SPC charts

As mentioned above, a frequency distribution provides a range within which nearly all of a process's future measures are likely to fall. That is, how a process behaved in the past is a reasonable predictor of how it will behave in the future.

Using this knowledge, Shewhart developed the concept of a control chart. Flipping a frequency distribution curve on its side and plotting individual observations from a process over time is the first step in creating a control chart. Each time you plot a point, you are really saying to yourself, "Is it reasonable that the random nature of this process could be producing this new measured result?" Adding the upper and lower control limits defines the specification range of the process and allows one to differentiate random cause variation from assignable variation. Adding these elements results in an SPC chart, as shown in Figure 46.

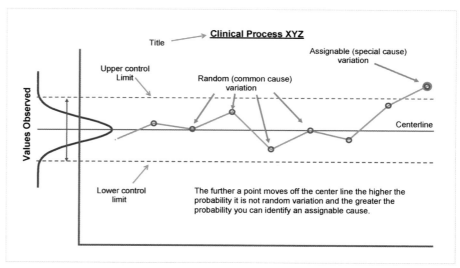

Figure 46: Statistical process control chart

A control chart is made up of several elements. The title briefly describes the information displayed in the chart. The y-axis shows the scale of the measurement for variables (numeric) data or the count (frequency) or percentage of occurrence of an event for attribute data. The x-axis displays the chronological order in which the data were collected.

In healthcare, control limits are generally set at a distance of Three Sigma above and Three Sigma below the centerline. They indicate variation from the centerline and are calculated by using the actual values plotted on the control chart graphs. The centerline is drawn at the average, or mean, value of all the plotted data. The centerline generally denotes the expected outcome or output of a given process. Thus, the centerline can also be said to represent the process capability of a process. If a process is improved, one can expect the centerline — and, therefore, the process capability — to move closer to the ideal or optimal outcome for the process.

Applying SPC charts

SPC charts are useful for monitoring process variation over time, differentiating between assignable cause and random cause variation, identifying and eliminating unwanted assignable variation, and assessing the effectiveness of changes on improving a process, as shown in Figure 47.

Figure 47 displays a key goal of a control chart — achieving and maintaining process stability. Process stability is defined as a state in which a process has displayed a certain degree of consistency in the past and is expected to continue to do so in the future. This consistency is characterized by a stream of data falling within control limits that are generally based on plus or minus three standard deviations (Three Sigma) of the centerline. Less stringent control limits (closer to the centerline) can result in misinterpreting random cause variation as assignable cause variation. Control limits represent the limits of variation that should be expected from a process in a state of statistical control. When a process is in statistical control, any variation is the result of random causes that affect the entire process in a similar way.

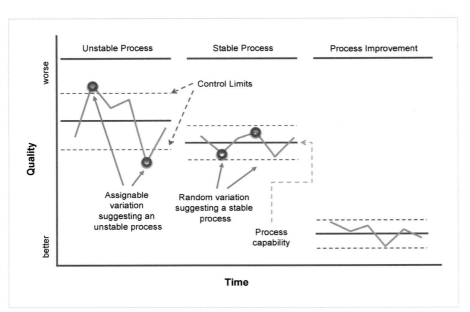

Figure 47: Use of control charts

As outlined above, control charts typically include data from a process plotted over time, with a centerline representing the median and upper and lower control limits that are typically set at three standard deviations from the mean (Three Sigma). When data points appear within the control limits, the process is exhibiting random variation and therefore is considered to be in statistical control, or stable.

On the other hand, control charts can also be used to identify assignable causes of variation. There are several guidelines that indicate when a signal of assignable cause variation has occurred on a control chart. The foremost rule is that a data point appears outside the control limits. Since the control limits are usually set at three standard deviations from the mean, one can state that for a process that is producing normally distributed data, the probability of a measurement appearing outside the control limits (upper or lower limit) is about 4 or 5 out of 1,000.

Several other rules have also been promoted to help identify assignable cause variation based on patterns of data points occurring within the control limits. While there is disagreement about some of the guidelines, three rules are widely recommended:

- A run of eight (some prefer seven) or more points on one side of the centerline.

- Two out of three consecutive points appearing beyond two standard deviations on the same side of the centerline (i.e., two-thirds of the way toward the control limits).

- A run of eight (some prefer seven) or more points all trending up or down.

Tampering

One of the most important concepts that came out of Shewhart's work was the concept of tampering. Tampering occurs when a manager uses techniques for managing assignable variation to deal with random variation. If you tamper, you effectively broaden the frequency distribution and increase the defect rate of a process. Tampering always increases the amount of variation and increases the defect rate. Avoiding tampering is particularly important in healthcare because it can worsen patient outcomes and lead to harm.

> "Tampering always increases the amount of variation and increases the defect rate. Avoiding tampering is particularly important in healthcare because it can worsen patient outcomes and lead to harm."

In a classic article published in "Medical Care" in 1991, Dr. Berwick used a clinical example to illustrate the risks of tampering:

> Brian was a year-old patient admitted to the hospital with possible osteomyelitis. It was only "possible" because, although the clinical picture and a bone scan in an outlying hospital were consistent with the diagnosis, no organism had been recovered from Brian's blood- stream. Antibiotic therapy had been started on an empirical basis, but Brian had continued to spike fevers for a week after treatment began. He was transferred for further evaluation. The clinical question of greatest importance was this: Did Brian, indeed, have osteomyelitis, with an organism sensitive to the current antibiotic or was a different process operating, perhaps osteomyelitis with a resistant organism or maybe another disease, such as lymphoma?
>
> The diagnostic strategy included careful observation. Over the next 14 days, Brian was, indeed, observed, and among the observations made were measurements of his temperatures. During that period, his antibiotic regimen was changed three times, he underwent multiple imaging tests, and had both a bone biopsy and a bone marrow biopsy. During those 14 days, Brian had 100 separate temperature measurements recorded in his chart. Those 100 measurements appeared, in fact, on 22 separate pages of nursing notes.
>
> Show this list to Walter Shewhart, and he would feel quite at home. A measurement system exists, which reports on an important process variable and is placed at the disposal of "operators" (in Shewhart's language) who are to make adjustments based on the measurement. In a manufacturing process, the adjustments would involve dials and levers; here they involve modifications of antibiotics and testing strategies.
>
> When Shewhart studied systems like this at Bell Telephone Laboratories, he discovered that the information was not being used very well. The "operators" of the gauges and machines in fact varied greatly in the ways in which they responded to the information. They varied among themselves, and even a single decision maker varied over time in his or her own apparent rules of action. Operators often overreacted, making adjustments in settings in response to variation that, through the lens of Shewhart's statistical understanding, was simply random. In over adjusting, they produced more variation than they started with. They actually made the system less reliable, instead of more reliable, an effect that Deming was later to call 'tampering" but that Shewhart simply called 'errors of Type I.'

Managers, too, tampered. Unable to understand the underlying causes of the variation they saw, managers changed systems in response to variations that were merely random or not caused by the system in the first place, thereby adding complexity but doing no good. Systems got more and more complex, costs rose, and quality suffered.

Does this sound like a modern hospital or not? What are the rules of action that allow a group of six house officers and five consultants to adjust antibiotic dosages based on a stream of 101 temperature measurements? Based upon what statistical theory do they work? Are the changes in management, e.g., hold the antibiotics, start the antibiotics, change the antibiotics, draw a new culture, biopsy the bone, biopsy the marrow, fight the fever with acetaminophen, observe the fever without acetaminophen, systematic interventions on meaningful variations clearly interpreted; or do the clinicians, too, tamper by misinterpreting the signals as noise or the noise as signals' How much of the effort that is poured into the patient, how much of the money, would Shewhart show to be waste, waste that is exactly equivalent to waste the machine tool operator makes when, standing before his or her gauges, he or she adjusts lever after lever in response to meaningless, random, common cause variation?

How much tampering of this exact kind, the kind Shewhart noticed and set about to help others notice, eats into the day-to-day work of clinical management in medical care? No one really knows. The cost could be enormous. Clinicians, flooded today with the results of measurement upon measure- merit, undoubtedly face serious risks of misunderstanding variation in what is being measured.

Think about the ramifications. Where do clinicians measure and respond clinically based on that measurement? The list is endless. Measure prothrombin times and change anticoagulants. Measure oxygen tensions and change respirator settings. Measure fever and change antibiotics. Measure blood pressure and change antihypertensive. Measure leukocytes and change chemotherapies. Measure pain and change analgesia. Measure electrolytes and change IV fluids. Measure and change, measure and change.

In fact, the process of managing data in health care has not changed much at all, even as the volume and complexity of those data have grown by orders of magnitude during this century.

Physicians need not be frightened of trying to master an understanding of variation in these terms.[81]

Using SPC and control charts to better understand variation and to more effectively manage processes is foundational to effective quality improvement in any industry, including healthcare. In this regard, Shewhart's pioneering work and its subsequent application to quality improvement by Deming has proven revolutionary in our ability to understand variation and improve processes. We owe a great deal of gratitude to Shewhart for his revolutionary ideas. In the same article, Dr. Berwick recognized Shewhart's contribution as follows:

> Walter Shewhart was a student of, above all, causes. He believed that results in complex systems did not just happen but were the consequences of lawful relationships; maybe it was because he was a physicist that he chose to interpret production that way. He believed that, properly analyzed, experience in real causal systems could teach a great deal about those systems, and he devoted much of his professional career to developing methods through which the study of variation in measured results could teach the observer about the causal systems that led to those results. If he had been a physician, he would have been called an applied epidemiologist, or a clinical researcher — and a master at it.[81]

Now that we have reviewed variation and how it applies to quality improvement, we will turn our attention to a conversation about how we use data in quality improvement to maximize clinician engagement and outcomes. For those who would like to learn more about variation and statistical process control, please read Appendix B.

A thoughtful approach to improvement — focus on better care, not people

Once the care process families are prioritized, an organization can focus its attention on improving them. This starts with how to appropriately use data in quality improvement.

> "
> Walter Shewhart was a student of, above all, causes. He believed that results in complex systems did not just happen but were the consequences of lawful relationships ...
> "

How do we measure outcomes? How do we determine which are good outcomes and which are not? This brings us back to the concept of variation. A good outcome is generally viewed as one that represents the optimal outcome for a given process. That is, it represents best practice in the eyes of reasonable clinicians. Once we have determined the ideal outcome, the performance of clinicians can be plotted on a frequency distribution. Using the frequency distribution, we can then determine which outcomes represent reasonable, or random, variations from the norm and which represent assignable cause variations, or so-called outliers.

In Figure 48, the x-axis shows variability in outcomes for a clinical process, with poor outcomes on the left and excellent outcomes on the right for a care process family. The y-axis on each grid shows the number of cases for each outcome. When you see the first grid your initial reaction might be to target only the cases with poor outcomes. That is, focus on the outcomes that deviate far enough from the norm that they are deemed unacceptable. This is called punishing the outliers, or cutting off the tail. When you use this approach, the outliers usually improve barely enough to meet the new minimum standard. Meanwhile, the acceptable outcomes — which constitute most of a hospital's cases — do not budge.

The goal of quality improvement is to move everyone in the direction of continuously better care. That is, to move the centerline of the outcome frequency distribution and the entire bell-shaped curve toward an improved outcome. By definition, this approach will automatically identify any outliers (bad apples), but the focus is primarily on improving everyone's performance rather than focusing on those few bad apples. Outliers will either learn to improve or self-select out by demonstrating unwillingness to improve.

Thus, a more effective approach to improving a care process family is to narrow the curve (i.e., narrow the spread of the frequency distribution) and

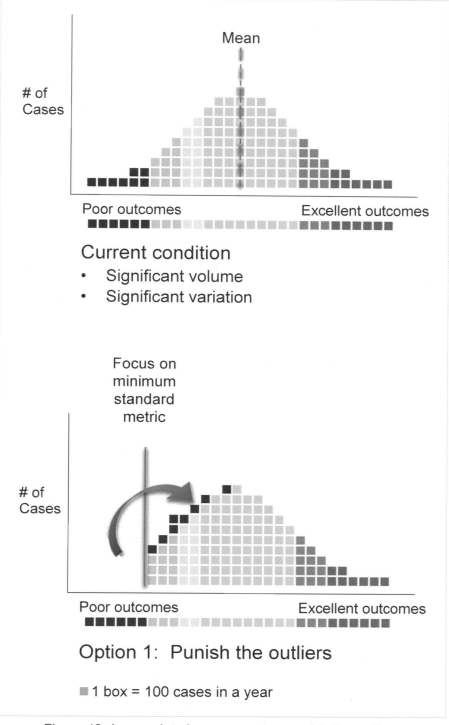

Figure 48: Approach to improvement — punish the outliers

move all cases closer to better outcomes, as seen in Figure 49. In order to achieve high-quality outcomes and reduce waste, one needs to focus on eliminating inappropriate variation (focus on processes) and documenting continuous improvement (focus on outcomes). This is illustrated in Figure 49 by a narrowing of the distribution of the curve (eliminating inappropriate variation) and the entire curve shifting to the right (improving outcomes).

Instead of focusing on the outliers, improvement teams identify evidence-based shared baselines and use them to reduce variation in all cases — a tactic known as inlier management. Inlier management improves outcomes across the board, producing a much greater overall impact.

Positive reinforcement has been demonstrated to be far more effective with people than a negative, judgmental approach. This is particularly true of clinicians, who generally pride themselves in being the best they can be for patients. While good data may demonstrate that some of them may be misguided in assessing the quality of the care they give, they still want to be the best they can be and are more likely to respond to a collaborative process that engages them in a continuous improvement journey. Even if physicians initially question the data, as they often will, it is okay. The very fact that they are questioning the data means the focus is on a data-driven assessment of the quality of care. Either the data will be proven wrong, in which case the data can be corrected, or the data will be proven correct, in which case reasonable clinicians will seek to improve.

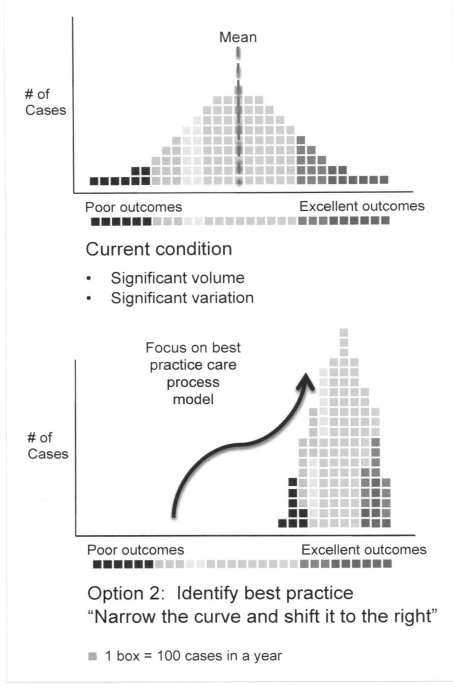

Figure 49: Approach to improvement — focus on better care

Now that we understand how to measure, differentiate and monitor different types of variation, as well as how data is best used in quality improvement, we can turn our attention to using data to identify meaningful patterns.

Figure 50 shows that frequency distributions can help an organization choose which care process families to focus on. Care process families that consume more resources and have more variability, such as those in quadrant 1, should be addressed first. Quadrant 2 shows care process families with high resource consumption but less variability than quadrant 1. Because the potential yield is lower, a network will want to avoid focusing on care process families where fewer resources are consumed, whether or not they have ample variation in outcomes, like those in quadrant 3, or minimal variation, like those in quadrant 4.

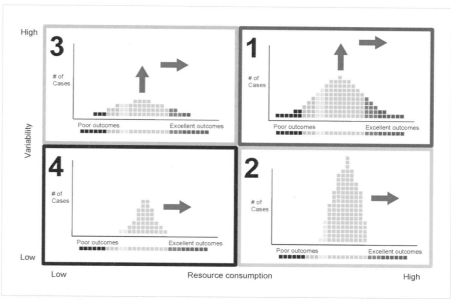

Figure 50: Improvement approach — prioritization
(View Appendix C for larger version)

Figure 51 illustrates one way of visualizing how care process families consume resources. This graph shows resources consumed on the x-axis and internal variation in cost on the y-axis. Remember that variability in cost often indicates clinical opportunity. The size of each bubble reflects the number of cases

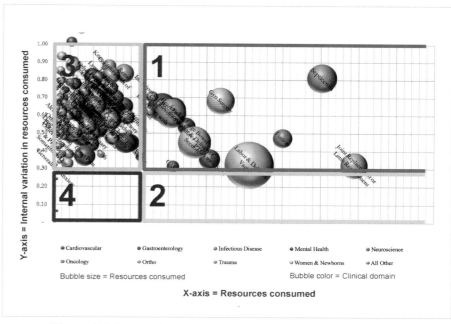

Figure 51: Internal variation versus resource consumption
(View Appendix C for larger version)

in that care process family. When we overlay our priority boxes, we can see which care processes to work on first. In this example, septicemia ranks very high in both resources consumed and internal variation. It also has a high case count. This makes it a great target for improvement efforts.

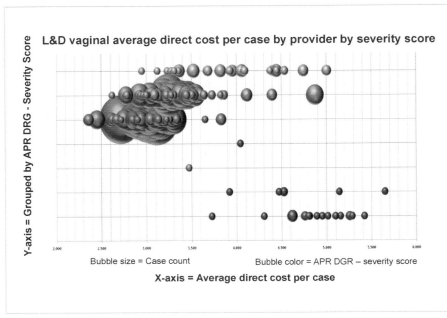

L&D vaginal average direct cost per case by provider by severity score

Y-axis = Grouped by APR DRG - Severity Score

Bubble size = Case count   Bubble color = APR DGR – severity score

X-axis = Average direct cost per case

Figure 52: Variation by provider example

Another data set to examine is variation by provider. Any time there is a wide variation in provider care, we have a high potential for standardization and cost savings. As one drills down to the physician level, significant variation in the cost of treating these patients by physician is apparent. In Figure 52 each bubble represents a different provider handling a specific set of labor and delivery patients. The size of the bubble represents the number of cases for that physician. The grid shows significant cost variation among physicians treating cases of the same severity. This probably occurs because they use different clinical approaches. If the physicians used a standardized, evidence-based process, all of the bubbles at the same severity level would be stacked on top of each other.

Up to this point, we have been talking mostly about clinical variation, but this alone does not account for all of the internal variation in cost. Variation in the data system — how clinicians define things, how they collect data and how they code activities — also contributes to variation. We may not be defining a care process the same way or collecting the data in the same way. This represents something that needs to be fixed in the name of data quality assurance.

Furthermore, variation will exist in operational processes just as it does in clinical processes. This type of variation will also impact costs. Organizations have the opportunity to identify and reduce variation in all areas. Assignable variation of any type — true differences in the way care is delivered by the providers or how operational processes are managed by staff — represent opportunities for standardizing care and operations to reduce variation from provider to provider and from department to department. Invariably, a reduction in variation has a desirable by-product of reducing costs.

Once we have unlocked an organization's data and made it readily accessible, prioritized the data to determine where to focus improvements and identified meaningful patterns in the data, we are in a better position to ignite change.

This completes the overview of the analytic system and its key components: unlocking the data, automating the distribution of data and discovering patterns in the data. Now that we've discussed the importance of measurement and the benefits of a strong analytic system, it is time to consider the deployment system. In the next chapter, we will discuss the organizational work that allows organizations to capitalize on the data they have unlocked, automated and begun to use in the analytic system. We will learn about team structures, roles, fingerprinting, implementation and other elements of effective deployment in chapter 5.

5 THE DEPLOYMENT SYSTEM: STANDARD ORGANIZATIONAL WORK

In chapter 4, we discussed the steps an organization can take to establish an analytic system. In this chapter, we will focus on the deployment system — an essential component in achieving scalable and sustainable quality improvement, improved clinical outcomes and patient experience, and reduced costs.

In this chapter, we will explore the importance of having appropriately resourced, permanent teams — teams that are backed by sound process improvement methods and a responsive analytic system. By the end of this chapter you will be able to identify the essential teams and their key interactions, explain the benefits of using an iterative, or Agile, approach for improvement and understand how to leverage the organization's analytic system to accelerate Lean process improvement.

These objectives are based on the three deployment system components illustrated in Figure 53:

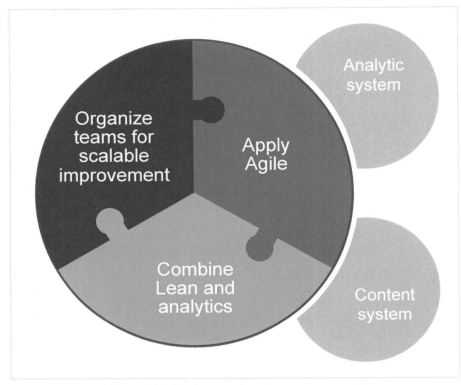

Figure 53: Deployment system components

- Organizing teams for scalable improvement

- Applying Agile principles to clinical quality improvement

- Combining Lean principles and analytics for sustainable gains

We will review each of the components in-depth. But first, let's turn our attention to some general principles regarding organizational readiness, the key role leaders play in change, and the importance of understanding and accounting for cultural values.

Chapter 5.1 — Key elements of organizational readiness

Successfully improving clinical quality outcomes and streamlining operations requires a strong organizational commitment and changes in culture, organizational structure, staff education and workflow processes. Consequently, as an organization embarks on a major quality improvement journey, it is important to assess the organization's readiness for change.

A readiness assessment helps an organization measure how prepared it is to accept change. An assessment will help the organization predict how change may impact staffing and how it will, or will not, affect clinical performance on the front lines of care. Results from a readiness assessment will also help shape an organization's approach to quality improvement initiatives.

To conduct a thorough readiness assessment, an organization needs to evaluate its culture, leadership styles, performance, processes and assets available to support major change. There are a variety of resources available to help healthcare organizations assess their readiness for change and create effective teams.[82, 83] An example of a readiness assessment tool used by Health Catalyst can be found at www.healthcatalyst.com/go/readiness-assessment-tool.

By completing a readiness assessment, an organization can identify needs and develop a change management plan. The readiness assessment can also help identify barriers that may impede progress and strengths that can be used to support a quality improvement program.

The role of senior leaders

A key component of an organization's readiness for change is the commitment of senior leaders — leaders who visibly lead the change and provide the resources to successfully implement change. First, senior leaders need to ensure that quality improvement initiatives are aligned with the organization's mission and strategic goals. Leaders also need to devote personal time and attention to the change initiative, be willing to invest in quality improvement, pay for the involvement of clinical opinion leaders, provide support resources (i.e., information technology, analytical resources, quality improvement expertise and facilitators), provide the necessary analytic system and deliver the education and training necessary for success.

> "A key component of an organization's readiness for change is the commitment of senior leaders — leaders who visibly lead the change and provide the resources to successfully implement change."

The learning organization

The importance of using data primarily for learning rather than for judgment or accountability was discussed in chapter 4. The concept of the learning organization, however, goes beyond the appropriate use of data.

In his well-known book "The Fifth Discipline: The Art and Practice of the Learning Organization," Peter Senge describes a learning organization as an organization "where people continually expand their capacity to create the results they truly desire, where new and expansive patterns of thinking are nurtured, where collective aspiration is set free, and where people are continually learning to see the whole together."[84]

Organizational research over the past two decades has revealed three broad factors that are essential for organizational learning and adaptability: a supportive learning environment, concrete learning processes and practices, and leadership behavior that provides reinforcement.[85] The characteristics of a learning organization are shown in Figure 54.

Organizational learning is strongly influenced by the behavior of the organization's leaders. If leaders actively question and listen to employees, and encourage dialogue and debate, people in the organization are motivated to learn. If leaders signal the importance of spending time on identifying problems, transferring knowledge and assessing project results, learning is likely to flourish. When people in power demonstrate through their own behavior a willingness to entertain alternative points of view, employees feel empowered to offer new ideas and options.

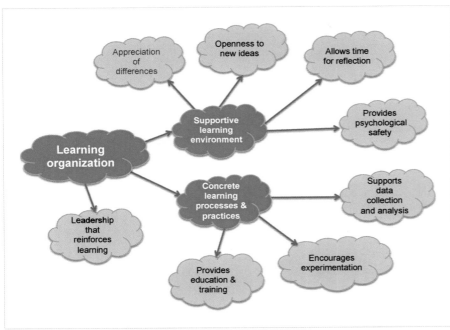

Figure 54: Characteristics of a learning organization

A learning organization is one that is able to change its behaviors and mindsets as a result of experience. Such organizations build environments that promote learning and leadership at all levels — so-called distributed leadership. These organizations seek to be accountable and encourage individuals and teams within the organization to accept responsibility for their actions. Learning organizations are characterized by a strong sense of individual responsibility. Accountability is clear, strong and widespread throughout the organization. People throughout a learning organization act as responsible agents working toward a shared vision, exploring possibilities and taking on initiatives that align with the organization's strategic initiatives. This is typically achieved through strong relationships and peer support rather than by mandates.

By fostering a learning environment, organizations are able to inform their business strategy by taking advantage of distributed intelligence throughout the system. Learning organizations fully engage internal stakeholders by responding to their issues. They change the behavior of the organization by changing the mindsets and attitudes of individuals within the organization. Finally, they integrate principles and practices of sustainability into the organization's culture.

Organizational learning is more than individual learning. It arises from the interaction of individuals and teams, but it is more than the separate contributions of individuals and teams. Organizational learning occurs when individuals and teams work together throughout the system.

To succeed, organizational learning needs the right environment, one that allows time for reflection on past actions and outcomes and where members are prepared to accept some unpleasant realities. Learning organizations cannot tolerate a blame culture where mistakes are unacceptable. A learning environment makes a distinction between mistakes that result from irresponsibility and lack of forethought and those that follow genuine explorations of a new idea or a new way of thinking or working. If individuals and teams are encouraged to be innovative, the organization needs to supply them the psychological safety to explore alternatives and to take well-reasoned risks. Learning organizations accept the reality that not all projects will succeed, and failures are not mistakes. Instead, they are viewed as learning opportunities. Failed projects are simply part of the search to find new, innovative products, services, processes and ways of working.

The learning organization also supplies the necessary education and training to enable individuals and teams to be successful, as well as the analytic system that provides the data-driven insights necessary to support continuous improvement.

> The benefits of the learning organization are well documented. Learning organizations maintain high levels of innovation and remain competitive — and they are better able to respond to external pressures.

The benefits of the learning organization are well documented. Learning organizations maintain high levels of innovation and remain competitive — and they are better able to respond to external pressures.[86] These organizations acquire the knowledge to better align resources with customer needs, and they are able to improve outcomes at all levels of the organization. Finally, they exhibit and tolerate a greater rate of organizational change.[87] Those interested in reading more about a learning healthcare organization are encouraged to read the IOM reports on the topic.[88, 89]

Creating a culture of quality and safety

A key subset of a healthcare organization's readiness is establishing a culture focused on promoting quality and patient safety. Peter Drucker, a renowned American business management consultant, is purported to have once said, "Culture eats strategy for lunch." There is truth in this statement. The best organizational strategies, including quality improvement strategies, can flounder if leaders do not pay attention to the organization's culture. Leaders that do not pay attention to culture risk failure.

Organizational culture includes the shared beliefs, experiences and expectations of people within an organization. In order to drive a major quality improvement initiative forward, the organization's culture must embrace a nonpunitive, mutually supportive environment. Clinicians and staff members who share the organization's vision are more willing to adapt to change. If an organization's existing culture does not support change, work must be done to transform clinicians' and employees' perceptions before moving forward with the initiative. The organization's leadership team needs to build a culture that promotes learning, effective teamwork and patient-centered care.

Senior leaders hold the ultimate responsibility for creating and maintaining a culture of safety and quality throughout the organization. Safety and quality thrive in an environment that supports open communication, teamwork and respect among all caregivers, regardless of their position. Leaders must demonstrate their commitment to quality and safety and set clear expectations for everyone in the organization. Effective leaders encourage teamwork and create structures, processes and programs that allow this positive culture to flourish. From the governing board to the front line, it is important to broaden knowledge of — and commitment to — quality and patient safety.

When this cultural work is done well, clinicians and staff recognize that quality and patient safety are valuable to the organization. It is important for clinicians and staff to be engaged in defining system-wide goals and demonstrating how safety and quality improvement initiatives tie into the organization's strategy. By focusing the organization's mission on quality improvement and safety, aligning quality improvement and safety aims with system-wide goals, and making staff aware of current performance, an organization's senior leaders can help establish the environment required for successful quality improvement.

Leadership practices unique to promoting patient safety

While leadership is critical to any quality improvement initiative, there are some leadership practices that are unique to promoting patient safety. Leadership is a critical element in any successful patient safety program and is not something that can be delegated. Only senior leaders can productively direct efforts to foster the culture and commitment required to address the underlying causes of harm. Healthcare leaders have used several established practices to effectively advance their organization's patient safety efforts.

One of these leadership best practices is "walk rounds." Ideally, these rounds occur weekly, pairing the patient safety officer (PSO) with a senior member of the executive team (such as the CEO or COO). Typically, these rounds consist of brief (30-minute) visits to individual units or clinics to hear safety concerns from front-line caregivers. During these rounds, leaders should ask specific questions to promote discussions around topics relevant to a safety culture, such as asking about situations when it is difficult to speak up. Leaders might include examples from their own personal experience that demonstrate situations when it was difficult to question someone in a leadership position.

Safety rounds provide an opportunity to remind staff of leadership's commitment to, and support for, speaking up and constantly looking for situations that could result in patient harm, such as a reluctance to speak up because of authority gradients.

The term "authority gradient" was first defined in aviation when it was noted that pilots, copilots and other flight crew members may not communicate effectively in stressful situations if there is a significant difference in experience, perceived expertise or authority. A number of aviation and other industrial incidents have been attributed, in part, to authority gradients.

> Safety rounds provide an opportunity to remind staff of leadership's commitment to, and support for, speaking up and constantly looking for situations that could result in patient harm, such as a reluctance to speak up because of authority gradients.

Nowhere was the impact of these authority gradients more apparent than in a Korean Airlines incident. Between 1970 and 2000 a number of high-profile airplane crashes plagued Korean Airlines. Detailed analyses of these incidents concluded that aspects of Korean national culture, such as respect for authority, played a significant role in crashes because lower-level crewmembers refrained from challenging a captain's decisions. A crash that occurred in 1999 is illustrative of this. Because South Korean military discipline permeated Korean airline cockpits, the co-pilot and a flight engineer on a Korean Air Boeing 747 flight did not insist that the pilot abort the landing until just 6 seconds before a crash that killed 228 people — even after altitude alarms sounded in the cockpit.

The authority problem is not unique to Korean Airlines. Veteran pilots and airline industry experts identified similar problems in airlines throughout the world, and many fatal crashes were attributed to the problem before speaking up was instituted as a cultural norm among flight crew members worldwide.

The concept of the authority gradient and its role in patient harm was first introduced into healthcare in the IOM's "To Err Is Human" report. As they do in many industries, power gradients can exist in healthcare, and the failure of clinical team members to speak up when potential harm situations are apparent can be devastating for patients.

> As they do in many industries, power gradients can exist in healthcare, and the failure of clinical team members to speak up when potential harm situations are apparent can be devastating for patients.

Similarly, examples of how to address disruptive behavior or a physician who is opting out of a safety protocol might be discussed on walk rounds. Specific issues discovered on rounds should be brought back to the organization's Patient Safety Committee, and a closed feedback loop should be created where staff can learn that their suggestions made during rounds were heard and appropriately acted upon. Using real patient stories to highlight patient safety topics is an important part of the cultural change strategy as well.

Paul Batalden, MD, emeritus professor at the Dartmouth Institute, has said, "Every system is perfectly designed to get the results it gets." Leaders who participate in walk rounds need to remember the truth of Dr. Batalden's observation. The aim of these walk rounds is not to fix people, but rather to fix processes.

It is also important to promote unit-based patient-safety problem solving. An environment in which unit-based problem solving is the norm, not the exception, should characterize individual care units. Safety should be a routine part of unit meetings and a key responsibility of unit and clinic managers. Activities in the unit should include sharing stories of harm and near misses, tackling problems, sharing best practices, distributing educational materials, creating awareness of regional and system-wide initiatives, and identifying potential opportunities for improvement and sources of harm for the hospital or regional patient safety officer.

Patients are also a valuable source of patient safety information. Walk rounds should include visiting directly with patients and their families. Asking questions such as, "Have you noticed if caregivers are washing their hands?" can be very enlightening and provide a powerful reminder to staff of the importance of involving patients in all we do.

There can be a tendency to focus on the positive. Because leaders may gravitate to high-performing care units, they should use surveys to identify units where they are most needed. Adopt-a-unit or clinic programs can be a powerful way to promote a safety culture. In these programs, low-performing units are visited more frequently and given additional attention by safety leadership. For instance, if the culture surveys indicate that nurses on a specific unit feel incident reports result in punitive action, discussions with unit managers need to be initiated to ensure that a learning culture is maintained.

Disruptive behavior that intimidates others can reduce morale, increase staff turnover and negatively impact both safety and patient care. Leaders must address disruptive behavior regardless of where it occurs. This includes management, clinical and administrative staff and independent practitioners. Leaders must make it clear that disruptive or dismissive behavior should be reported and will be taken seriously. Organizational leaders need to work with the medical staff leadership team to ensure they are addressing disruptive or dismissive behavior as seriously as they address poor clinical outcomes.

Healthcare arguably has the most well-educated and committed workforce in the world. The vast majority of clinicians get up every day wanting to do their best for the patients they serve. However, as intelligent, well-educated and committed as they are, clinicians do not necessarily understand the need for change, the quality improvement concepts and tools required to change, or their role in leading change.

> To drive quality improvement and patient safety forward, you have to have the passionate engagement of clinicians — healthcare's smart cogs.

To drive quality improvement and patient safety forward, you have to have the passionate engagement of clinicians — healthcare's smart cogs. Experiences in other industries have demonstrated that spreading new, innovative ideas can be accomplished by paying attention to the so-called opinion leaders that exist in all groups of people of sufficient size. The same approach works in healthcare.

In 1962, Everett Rogers, a professor of communication studies, published a book entitled "Diffusion of Innovations."[90] In the book, Rogers suggests that diffusion is a process by which innovation is communicated and spread throughout an organization or social system. The book suggests four main elements that influence the spread of a new idea: innovation, communication channels, time and a social system. The process of diffusion is heavily dependent on human capital because in order to sustain itself, an innovation must be widely adopted. Rogers suggests that within the rate of adoption, there is a point at which the innovation achieves critical mass. Rogers also identified five categories of adopters: innovators, early adopters, early majority, late majority and laggards. These categories and their characteristics are illustrated in Figure 55.

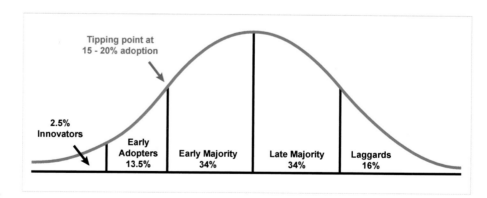

Figure 55: Rogers diffusion of innovation model

Innovators tend to be more cosmopolitan and open to new ideas. They try new ideas more readily. Like innovators, early adopters tend to be opinion leaders. While they may not initially embrace a new innovation, they are quick to adopt new ideas that are credible. As long as the innovators and early adopters show the way, the early majority will accept new innovations and willingly legitimize the innovation. The late majority tends to be more skeptical, but if others are willing to prove that an innovation works, they are willing to eventually follow suit. Laggards tend to be skeptical and accept new ideas only with great reluctance. Many laggards will die or retire without accepting new innovations even when they are clearly accepted by others.

It has been shown that the tipping point or critical mass for broad adoption of a new innovation tends to occur when about 20 percent of the workforce embraces new innovations. At that point innovators and early adopters (i.e., opinion leaders) have already embraced the innovation.

All clinical teams have opinion leaders. They represent Rogers innovators and early adopters. Organizational leaders need to identify these opinion leaders among their clinicians and develop a strategy to inform and engage them. Once these opinion leaders are engaged, they will influence the rest of the medical and nursing staff to more readily embrace new ideas and innovations.

Chapter 5.2 — Organizing permanent teams for scalable improvement

Organizational teams that can drive scalable improvement are one component of a deployment system. To improve deployment systems, an organization needs to start by establishing permanent teams that take ownership of the quality, cost and patient satisfaction associated with care delivery. An organization also needs to organize team structures, provide training on roles, allow teams to design their own solutions and ensure improvement is implemented consistently. Encouraging clinicians to design new ways of doing things creates a sense of ownership in the solutions they deploy.

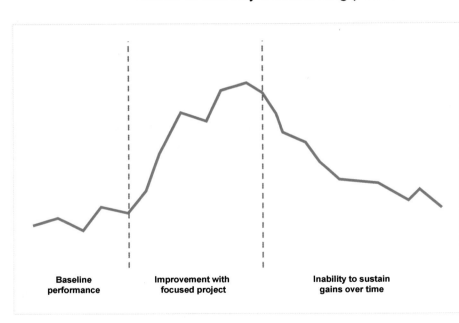

Baseline performance   **Improvement with focused project**   **Inability to sustain gains over time**

Figure 56: Outcome of a typical deployment system

Organizations often deploy teams when they need to make a change, but few do it in a manner that supports scalable and sustainable gains. As a result, they often enjoy temporary success followed by a return to baseline performance. Common characteristics of such teams — as depicted in Figure 56 — include being temporarily assigned, receiving little or no support from members of the organization's technical team, approaching the work like a project with a defined beginning and end and having no access to an analytic system.

Some quality departments review regulatory quality reports and then form a SWAT team to go to work on the biggest problem. They focus intensely on that problem until it is adequately "fixed" and then move to the next problem. This strategy has a tendency to make care delivery departments feel like they don't own the care improvement process.

Clinical process improvement is the responsibility of front-line workers working in partnership with quality departments. Because front-line caregivers understand the process of care delivery best, they are best suited to own the responsibility to eliminate waste and improve existing processes. This is where continuous improvement actually happens. Quality departments also play an important role by providing support to front-line caregivers as the caregivers improve processes, spread improvement practices across a healthcare system and address regulatory needs.

Elements of an effective deployment system

When an organization begins to develop their deployment system, we recommend that they assemble a few essential teams: executive team, guidance teams, clinical implementation teams and work groups. All of these teams have several things in common. They are permanent, they support related care process families, and they integrate clinical and technical experts. The makeup and role of each team is described below — and team interactions are illustrated in Figure 57.

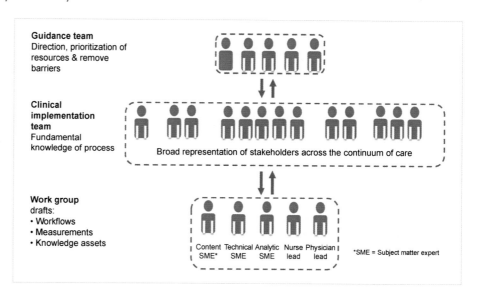

Figure 57: Team interactions

- ⊙ The executive team is accountable for and prioritizes all clinical quality initiatives across the healthcare organization. Team members could include people with job titles such as CEO, CMO, CNO, CIO, CMIO, etc. Guidance teams report their progress to this team.

- ⊙ Guidance teams are accountable for clinical quality across the continuum of care in a specific domain (e.g., Women and Children's or Cardiovascular). These teams consist primarily of clinicians and administrative leaders. Their role is to select goals within their clinical area (or domain), prioritize work, allocate resources, foster communication and eliminate barriers to ensure successful, continuous process improvement.

Guidance teams assign accountability to clinical implementation teams (CITs) to improve care within a care process family.

- ⊗ Clinical implementation teams (CITs) are generally led by a physician and nurse and consist of front-line staff that has fundamental knowledge of each major activity within a care process family, such as heart failure, AMI, CABG, etc. These teams should have a broad representation (e.g., key clinics, hospitals, regions, etc.). Their role is to refine work group outputs and lead the implementation of process improvements. CITs generally create work group teams to perform the detailed work within a care process family.

- ⊗ Work groups are generally led by a physician and nurse subject matter expert and include content, analytics and technical experts. They may be led by a pharmacist, respiratory therapist, or a finance or lab director, depending on the type of improvement project. This team meets frequently to analyze processes and data and to look for trends and improvements. The work group's role is to develop Aim Statements, identify interventions, draft knowledge assets (e.g., order sets, patient safety protocols, etc.,), define the analytic system and provide ongoing feedback of the status of the care process improvement initiatives. Outputs from this team are taken to the CIT.

Effective leaders need to be identified for all of these teams. Team leaders should be selected based on their knowledge of the clinical or organizational process as well as their leadership, facilitation and communication skills. Clinical team members must also have a deep understanding of the care process that is being improved. The only individuals who really know how a process works are those that perform the process every day.

Clinical implementation team members have two additional responsibilities: they should use their knowledge to describe and improve the process and then share the improved process with their co-workers. It is not just what team members bring to the table, but what they bring back to the front line. Without team members that adequately understand a particular clinical process, it is unlikely that a process will be accurately defined using visual process tools (e.g., value stream maps, A3s, etc.), nor is it likely that the changes would be accepted by the clinicians who are ultimately impacted.

Now let's explore the typical sequence of interactions between these teams. Process changes, knowledge assets such order sets and patient safety protocols, and metrics are drafted within the work group. These items are reviewed and modified with the CIT. This feedback loop is referred to as fingerprinting. Fingerprinting happens in all the teams and helps establishes buy-in across the entire organization. Regular updates are provided from the

CIT to the guidance team.
Figure 58 displays the standard
organizational workflow.

A project example

In order to illustrate this
process, let's look at a
cardiovascular improvement
example.

The cardiovascular clinical
program guidance team
selects heart failure as the
highest priority opportunity
for improvement, based on
its being one of the largest
clinical processes in the
care delivery system and its
having a significant amount of

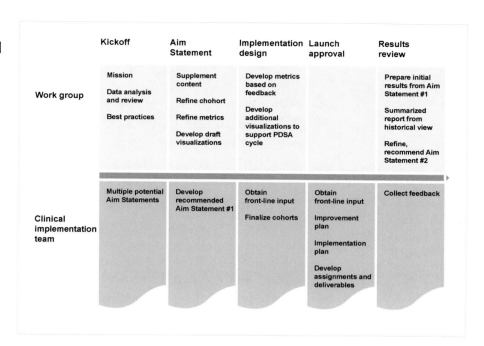

Figure 58: Standard organizational workflow
(View Appendix C for larger version)

variation when individual provider, clinic and hospital practices are compared.
The CIT explores the cohort of patients they are working with (i.e., the patient
population). The areas with significant disparity, lack of standardization and
variation in process and outcome results are highlighted and a decision is
made to focus on reducing 30-day heart failure readmissions. The CIT then
assigns a work group to review the information and focus on this problem.
The work group's first task is to understand the current state for preventing
30-day heart failure readmissions. They do this by reviewing current
processes (e.g., workflows, value stream maps). Next, they define a goal that
provides context for additional work. The goal they select is to reduce 30-day
heart failure by 3 percent in 2014. Next, the work group develops progressive
Aim Statements. The purpose of an Aim Statement is to establish clear
clinical improvement goals and integrate evidence-based practices in order
to standardize care. The CIT reviews the goal and Aim Statements to provide
input and direction. Examples of a progressive series of Aim Statements that
relate to the care process for heart failure might include the following:

> Aim Statement #1 — Data quality: By (specific date), establish a
> baseline for all cause 30-day readmission rates for patients found in
> the heart failure cohort and reconcile and validate against the previous
> year's baseline heart failure readmission rates by (date). This baseline
> will be used to measure before/after test results to determine what
> impact new interventions have on outcomes.

> Aim Statement #2 — Risk stratification: By (date), identify high-risk heart
> failure patients and establish a baseline for 30-day readmissions for

those patients. Extend the identification of these high-risk patients to a risk stratification model used to predict the likelihood of all cause 30-day readmission rates for heart failure patients.

- ⊗ Aim Statement #3 — Intervention: By (date), the heart failure team will develop one evidenced-based process metric (e.g., medication reconciliation, follow-up appointments, etc.) and one balance metric (e.g., ED admits, Observation days, etc.) that will have effect (X) on all cause 30-day readmission rates for high-risk patients. The intervention will be identified by the risk stratification model and baseline rates for the two measures will be established.

- ⊗ Aim Statement #4 — Intervention: Establish a medication reconciliation baseline and track compliance of heart failure medications (i.e., beta blocker, ACE or ARB) in order to achieve CMS compliance of (XX%) by (date).

- ⊗ Aim Statement #5 — Intervention: Establish a post-discharge follow-up phone call process baseline and track completion in order to achieve (XX%) compliance within (X) time after the patient is discharged by (specific date).

- ⊗ Aim Statement #6 — Post-discharge follow-up appointment: Establish a post-discharge follow-up appointment process baseline for a follow-up appointment within (X) days after discharge and track the scheduling of post-discharge follow-up appointments in order to achieve (XX%) compliance by (specific date).

When solutions are not obvious or intuitive, the healthcare system can pilot different interventions at separate hospitals, measure the outcomes and then compare the results within a specified timeframe. The best approach could be implemented system-wide, or the organization may take the best ideas from each approach and combine them into something entirely new.

Once a single approach is selected, it is launched system-wide. The CIT reviews the data on an ongoing basis with the guidance team, and the CIT and work group continue to work on new Aim Statements even as they continue monitoring progress on the existing ones. This allows the healthcare organization to sustain its gains while the teams begin work on new improvements. Taking this approach means there are permanent teams accountable for the ongoing performance of launched improvement initiatives. The result is sustained gains.

Tools for an effective deployment system

Organizational work can be challenging. Teams can benefit from a starter kit of tools that can help them with the role creation, team development and deployment process, rather than starting from scratch. As an example,

Health Catalyst provides an established framework and methodology, including a prebuilt starter kit. Figure 59 shows some of the materials in the starter kit, including team charters, job descriptions, physician contract templates, levels of compensation, job family grids, slide decks, handbooks, sample meeting agendas, deployment process outlines and sample project status reports.

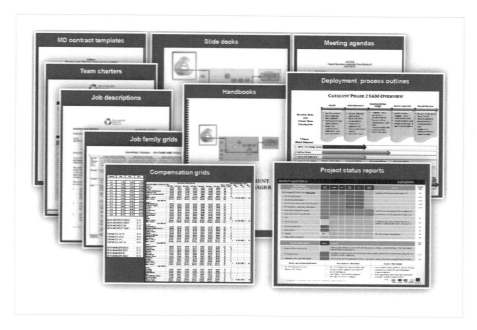

Figure 59: Sample starter tool kit

There are also a number of methods and techniques teams can leverage to be successful. For example, if teams are trying to generate a broad range of options based on expert opinion across a group, they might use brainstorming, multi-voting, or Nominal Group Technique tools (i.e., NGT or Delphi methods).

As teams use these tools, they should engage in data-driven problem solving. Managing and improving a process requires the right data, delivered in the right format, at the right time and to the right set of process experts. Accurate data allows teams to explain findings and suggest improvements to the front-line caregivers as they pursue input and acceptance. Combined with good data, the healthcare analytic visualizations convey the information in an easy-to-understand format that helps drive engagement and acceptance from front-line workers. Having said this, it is important to remember that there is a difference between having data that is good enough to support improvement and perfect data. Clinicians will rarely have perfect data, and insisting on perfect data can easily result in no progress in improving care. Recognizing when data is good enough to move on is a key attribute of success in process improvement.

There are several best practices that improvement teams can employ when launching a quality improvement initiative:

⦿ Executive commitment for permanent process improvement. Leadership must allocate the necessary resources to support permanent teams. Often this requires backfilling front-line positions because a senior front-line person may be called on to become a permanent member of the work group team. This can become a full-time position once multiple Aim Statements are underway. Of course, in smaller healthcare systems, this might not be feasible and these roles may need to remain part-time.

- Expert team members. Team members should be selected on the basis of who is needed rather than on who is available. Starting with the wrong team to address an issue can be a prescription for disaster.

- Training on quality improvement concepts. Teams need to be educated in basic quality improvement concepts before they begin an improvement project. While quality improvement concepts are not rocket science, a basic understanding is necessary for teams to be effective

- A defined charter. A well-crafted team charter provides a team the direction it needs to be successful in tackling the task it has been assigned.

- Established baseline data. Teams need to assure they have the baseline data they need when launching a new project.

- Understand root cause before defining a solution. Teams should avoid jumping to solutions before they have a thorough understanding of the root causes of a problem. It is a good practice to pilot a solution to determine how a solution will impact a problem before rolling the solution out across an organization.

- A clear idea of the goal they want to achieve. To solve a problem or to reach a goal, teams do not need to know all the answers in advance. But they must have a clear idea of the problem they want to solve or the goal they want to reach. This requires a concise Aim Statement. When creating an Aim Statement, it is useful to remember the SMART pneumonic.

> "Teams should avoid jumping to solutions before they have a thorough understanding of the root causes of a problem. It is a good practice to pilot a solution to determine how a solution will impact a problem before rolling the solution out across an organization."

SMART stands for specific, measurable, attainable, relevant and time-bound. Specific emphasizes the need for a goal that is clear and unambiguous. Measurable stresses the need for concrete criteria for measuring progress toward a goal's attainment. If a goal is not measurable, it is not possible to know whether a team is making progress. Attainable highlights the importance of goals that are realistic and achievable. While an attainable goal may stretch a team, the goal should not be extreme. That is, goals should be neither out of reach nor below standard performance, because these may turn out to be meaningless. Relevant implies the importance of choosing goals that matter. Time-bound underscores the importance of grounding goals within a timeframe and giving them a target date. A commitment to a deadline helps a team focus their efforts on completion on or before the due date. This part of the SMART goal criteria is intended to prevent goals from being overtaken by the day-to-day crises that invariably arise in an organization. A time-bound goal is intended to create a sense of urgency. Having a definite time frame will also help teams avoid making the Aim Statement too large in scope.

- ⊘ Defined problem-solving process. Teams need to follow a defined problem-solving process, such as Plan-Do-Study-Act (PDSA), to avoid wandering aimlessly.

- ⊘ Rapid cycle approach. Teams should take a rapid cycle approach. That is, craft well-defined Aim Statements that are achievable in a reasonable time frame, work through the PDSA cycle quickly, and seek a quick win. Then they should move on to something more complex and keep repeating the PDSA cycle.

- ⊘ Continuous process improvement. Teams should strive to mature and continuously improve their process as they address key challenges.

In thinking about the teams involved in deployment, it is important to remember that these teams meet regularly, both formally and informally. For example, the work group meets weekly. A few of the individual members of the work group may also meet informally on a daily basis. To maintain continuous improvement, they never stop meeting, and their improvement efforts are ongoing.

The best way to add clinical and business value when building an analytic system and deploying clinical improvement initiatives is to build incrementally and to use the system as you build it. This is achieved by using Agile principles, the second key component of the deployment system.

Chapter 5.3 — Applying Agile principles to improvement

In addition to forming the right teams, organizations also need to implement an Agile, or iterative, method that fosters continuous improvement. The Agile system for software development was developed about 15 years ago when a group of software developers gathered in the mountains above Salt Lake City and penned the Agile Manifesto, which argued for a better way of developing software. The manifesto emphasizes 4 core values: individuals and interactions over processes and tools; working software over comprehensive documentation; customer collaboration over contract negotiation; and responding to change over following a plan. One of those original developers, Alistair Cockburn, helped implement Agile principles at Intermountain Healthcare with great success.

A main principle of the Agile method is to start using a product while it is still being developed. To the uninformed, it may look as if developers are just winging it with no plan. However, in reality they are building incrementally with continuous feedback from front-line users, which allows the developers to add clinical and business value as the system is being completed.

To understand the Agile system, it helps to compare it to the traditional way of developing software — the so-called waterfall approach, as illustrated in Figure 60. In the waterfall approach, a project opens with requirements gathering, use cases and functional specifications, and then design specifications. Every step requires extensive documentation. Customers rarely see the product until the product is almost ready to launch, leaving little room to integrate user feedback and reaction to what has been built.

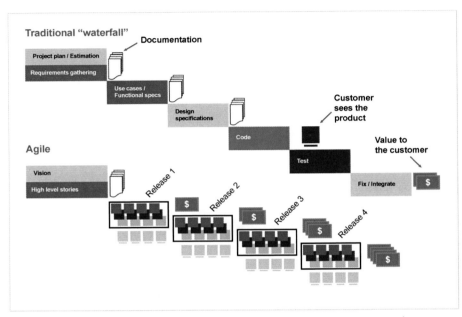

Figure 60: Traditional versus Agile development approach
(View Appendix C for larger version)

The Agile system takes a different approach. In a healthcare environment, developers quickly build high-level stories based on the problem clinicians are trying to solve. Within weeks, the work group can see what has been built, even if it is only a small component of the eventual product. This allows the work group to provide constant feedback to the developers. A weekly or bi-weekly rhythm is established where clinical end-users on the work groups view and critique the product, enabling the development team to make small adjustments and clarify what is needed. Clinicians on the work groups and clinical improvement teams play a vital role in this process because it provides them the opportunity to regularly interject their knowledge of the clinical process.

The Agile development system is a more effective way of delivering solutions, and it teaches clinicians and technical teams the value of working collaboratively. The benefits of the Agile approach and the limitations of the waterfall approach to development are illustrated in Figure 61 on page 111.

Using Agile principles has proven to be extremely valuable in helping to drive healthcare quality improvement. Clinical and technical teams need to build incrementally because clinicians do not always know what to measure at the outset. If they can see some data, react to it, adjust the measure and then repeat this process through multiple iterations, they eventually hone in on valuable metrics, valuable stratifications and important correlations in the data. During review loops, clinicians and developers look at graphical visualizations of the information, and clinicians request changes that developers can quickly make — sometimes even during the review meeting. This iterative and interactive process provides for more rapid development and ensures the delivered product meets clinicians' needs.

Chapter 5.4 — Combining Lean principles and analytics for sustainable gains

Once the right improvements teams are in place and an Agile approach to quality improvement has been adopted, organizations need to leverage their analytic system and Lean process improvement tools for immediate, automated feedback on performance and to ensure gains are sustained.

Benefits of the Agile approach to software development	Limitations of the waterfall approach to software development
Customers see software developments early and often	Customers see code only after months of work
Developers welcome changing requirements	Customer often says, "This is what I asked for but not what I want."
Businesspeople, clinicians and developers are motivated by trust and work together face-to-face and continuously	Software vendors push customers to specify their expectations in advance
Working software is the primary measure of progress	Strict milestones are established
Simplicity promotes sustainable development	Late changes mean additional charges
Team continually reflects and adjusts for a product everyone is happy with	Adversarial relationship between the people using and the people creating the software

Figure 61: Benefits of the Agile approach

Lean principles will be discussed in greater detail in chapter 6 (content system), but it is important to bring up some basic Lean concepts within the context of the analytic and deployment systems. By combining Lean with measurement, a team can identify and solve issues earlier because they have data and an automated analytic solution to measure improvements.

Lean processes focus on identifying value and eliminating waste. Using Lean techniques, improvement teams can quickly improve care. However, these teams are often challenged because they do not have access to the data to quickly identify the root cause of a problem or support sustainable gains. By integrating analytics, Lean improvement teams can identify root causes more rapidly. Improvement teams often rely solely upon observation. Improvement teams can observe past historical trends and pinpoint issues. By incorporating analytics, improvement teams have objective data that can direct them toward the key processes to observe.

When a work group first approaches a clinical process, it typically goes through a sequence where members map the process, identify wasteful steps in the process, identify ways of improving the process and create Aim Statements delineating specific improvement goals for the process. Once again, this is a way that front-line clinical experts on work groups and clinical improvement teams can interject their knowledge of clinical process into the improvement process.

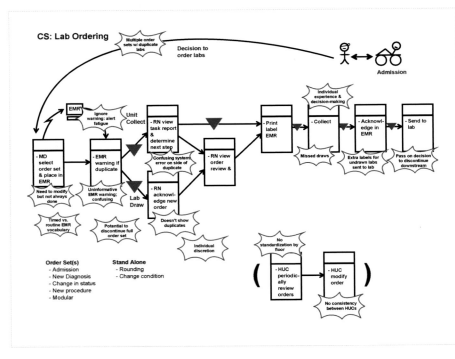

Figure 62: Using Lean to identify challenges
(View Appendix C for larger version)

A real-life example of this, created by a Health Catalyst client, is illustrated in Figure 62. The example is a value stream map of a lab ordering process. Value stream maps enable work group teams to identify all the major steps in a process. Once those steps are defined, teams can identify delays and waste in between each of the steps and determine ways to standardize and add value within each step. Value stream maps allow improvement teams to visually see the end-to-end process of how a service or product is delivered and better identify waste and improvement opportunities. The red storm clouds shown in Figure 62 identify potential problems and workarounds in the existing process. Let's look at a couple of the clouds to see how the improvement team was able to combine Lean principles with analytics to drive improvement.

The top red cloud identified duplicate lab orders as an issue. Duplicate order sets were recognized as a significant problem. When a lab was ordered twice, the patient was stuck twice, the lab performed the test twice and so on. The result was unnecessary pain for the patient and unnecessary cost. The improvement team had a hunch that duplicate order sets might be contributing to the duplicate labs.

The data that was available to the improvement team is shown in Figure 63. One order set stands out above the rest: potassium replacement. This order set accounts for 34 percent of the total duplicate labs ordered by the two largest specialties at the hospital — internal medicine and family practice. By quickly building a dashboard that showed all of the duplicate lab orders and the top duplicate lab orders, the team was able to quickly identify the root cause of the problem — and the single order set that was causing 34 percent of the duplicates. By eliminating just one order set that had a duplicate lab order connected with it, the improvement team immediately eliminated one-third of the problem.

Figure 62 contains another cloud burst on the value stream map that identified the issue of unclear duplicate definitions. The laboratory staff knew how to identify a duplicate lab because they could see the same test was being requested for the same patient. However, a physician may not have known about the duplicate lab because in certain ordering workflows, the overlapping orders were obscured.

The data that was available to this improvement team is shown in Figure 64. The data shared with the team showed 67 different reasons for lab cancellations, signifying real confusion around what constituted a duplicate. In fact, the reason for cancellation was not having a required documentation field in the ordering process. The result was that approximately 80 percent of the cancelled labs did not include a cancellation reason. The lab director saw that duplicate labs were the number one reason for cancellation and accounted for more than 95 percent of all cancelled labs. If her assumption was true, then the true level of duplicate labs was underreported in this data set. The data confirmed that duplicates were an issue, but it also showed that education around duplicates could drive improvement.

Cancelled Lab Procedures

Procedure Description	Procedure Description	
Procedure Code	POTASSIUM, SERUM	15.8%
	CREATININE EGFR	12.1%
	HEMOGLOBIN	11.7%
	BASIC METAB PROFILE	6.4%
	MAGNESIUM	6.2%
	TROPONIN I	5.3%
	PARTIAL THROMBOPLASTIN	4.3%
	PROTIME & INR	4.0%
	CBC	3.3%
	PLATELET COUNT	2.0%
	ELECTROLYTES	1.6%

Lab Cancellations

Reason	Reason	
Cancellation Code	Duplicate	33.8%
	Changed order	19.3%
	Discussed with RN	11.8%
	Other	8.9%
	See result narrative	4.3%
	Duplicate Floor Ordered	3.9%
	Error	3.8%
	Treatment ended	2.9%
	Patient condition	2.3%
	Clinician	1.6%
	Cancelled	1.5%

HIM Attending Provider

Specialty	Specialty	
Full Name	Internal Medicine	70.5%
	Family Medicine	29.5%
	Obstetrics/Gynecology	
	Pediatrics	
	Orthopedic Surgery	
	General Surgery	
	Psychiatry	
	Vascular Surgery	
	Neurosurgery	

Figure 63: Combining Lean and analytics: duplicate order sets

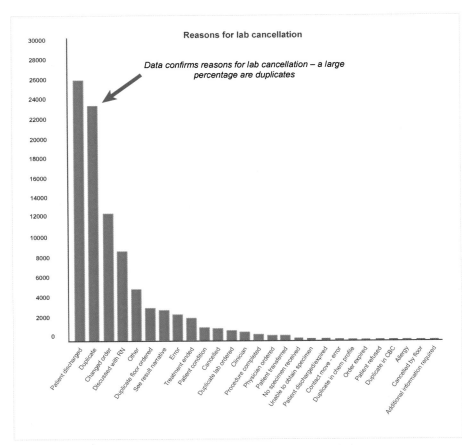

Figure 64: Lab cancellation example
(View Appendix C for larger version)

Clinicians may have been aware of the duplicate lab, but they failed to correct it at the source. Instead, they passed the order to the lab technician — the person who was most removed from the patient — to determine whether or not to cancel the lab test. The improvement team repeatedly asked the question, "Who is placing the duplicates? Can we see who it is by department and provider?"

The team received the data showing which department, specialty and provider was responsible for a duplicate lab order. Internal medicine physicians treating patients for septicemia ordered the vast majority of duplicate labs from department NMR 7SW.

The reasons for cancellation indicated that 40 percent of these canceled labs were because they were true duplicate orders. The data also showed the distribution of order sets that contributed to these duplicate labs. Potassium replacement accounted for 49 percent.

This example illustrates that the notion of physicians kicking the can down the road (i.e., delaying an important decision until a later, usually unspecified date) is not quite accurate. Broad, sweeping order sets appear to have contributed to a flawed workflow, again reinforcing the idea that a process is perfectly designed to get its results. Standardizing and refining order sets could be an appropriate area of focus for reducing duplicate lab orders.

These examples highlight the importance of integrating Lean processes into an improvement team's deployment strategy and also the importance of supporting those Lean processes with an analytic system. Not only can an improvement team pinpoint problems faster, they can also back them up with data and drill down to the root cause of the issues.

A healthcare organization with a healthy deployment system has the right teams in place to capture and use data, and applies an Agile approach and Lean principles in their improvement initiatives. The organization leverages an analytic platform to drive improved quality and reduced costs and is in a position to achieve scalable and sustainable improvement outcomes.

Next, we will turn our attention to the content system, the last of our three systems for effective care delivery.

6 THE CONTENT SYSTEM: STANDARD KNOWLEDGE WORK

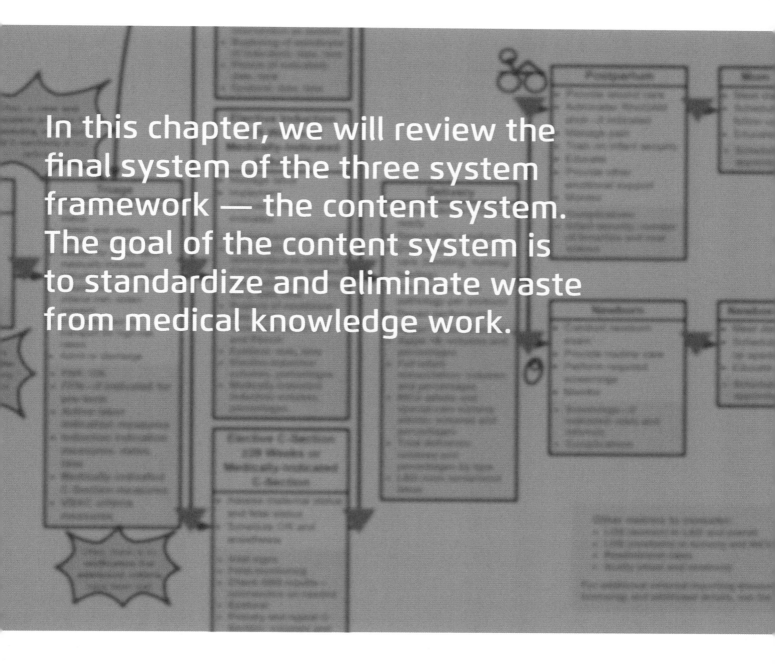

In this chapter, we will review the final system of the three system framework — the content system. The goal of the content system is to standardize and eliminate waste from medical knowledge work.

In chapter 4, we discussed the steps an organization can take to strengthen its analytic system in order to make data-driven decisions, and in chapter 5 we reviewed the characteristics of an effective deployment system which is essential to achieve scalable and sustainable quality improvement outcomes. In this chapter, we will review the final system of the three system framework — the content system.

The goal of the content system is to standardize and eliminate waste from medical knowledge work. Medical knowledge work is the process of taking today's best medical knowledge and having it become the standard in every day practice of most clinicians. Currently the process can take as long as 17 to 20 years to occur, as reported by the Agency for Healthcare Research and Quality (AHRQ).[72] This lag in the application of new knowledge is predominantly an outcome of a weak content system.

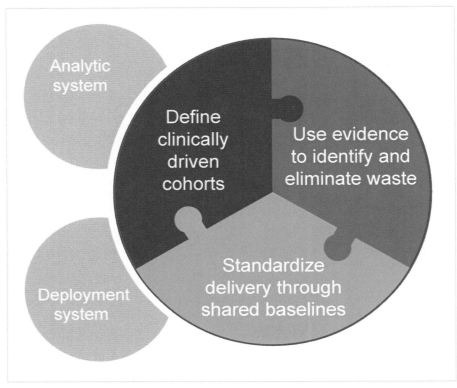

Figure 65: Content system components

By standardizing knowledge assets, such as order sets, intervention criteria, process flow maps and patient safety protocols, an organization can improve the speed at which new medical knowledge becomes everyday practice. This includes a consistent standard method for gathering evidence, evaluating that evidence and integrating it into care delivery.

An advanced clinical content system can decrease the lag time between the discovery of new knowledge and the standard application of that knowledge into clinical practice. As illustrated in Figure 65, the three major components of the content system include:

- ⊙ Defining a clinically driven patient cohort
- ⊙ Using evidence to identify and eliminate waste, and
- ⊙ Standardizing care through shared baselines

Together, these three components help healthcare systems ignite change by eliminating the non-value added, or wasteful activities, and hard wiring the most current evidenced-based activities into the care process. Consistent with Lean principles, this hard wiring enables clinicians to have an evidence-based, standardized way of delivering care that also supports deviation from the shared baseline when required for an individual patient. A content system allows organizations to achieve mass customization, where the variation in care is a result of the patient's condition and not in provider practice. Each of these content system components will be discussed in more detail, starting with the principles behind defining a clinically driven cohort.

By the end of this chapter you will understand how to identify cohorts of patients for quality improvement initiatives, how to use evidence to identify and eliminate waste, and the importance of standardizing care delivery through shared common baselines.

Chapter 6.1 — Defining clinically driven cohorts

A cohort is a group of patients with similar characteristics. There are three types of cohorts — chronic condition cohorts, episodic cohorts and procedural cohorts. A chronic condition cohort includes chronic conditions, such as asthma or diabetes. Episode centric cohorts revolve around a single episode of care like pregnancy that typically lasts nine months. An example of a procedural cohort could be an appendectomy. An appendectomy involves a one-time visit to the hospital and the episode of care requires minimal or no follow-up.

The first step is to identify what type of cohort you are dealing with. The procedural cohorts like appendectomy are reasonably straightforward: either you had an appendectomy or you haven't. Chronic conditions are more difficult to define since patients tend to go in and out of the cohort. For example, an asthma patient might get her asthma under control and have no further incidents for a year or more. But then, the asthma flares up when the patient gets a cold and develops a cough. It is important to develop the best cohort definition possible for these types of chronic conditions.

An example of defining an asthma cohort is illustrated in Figure 66. In this example, a work group created a simple initial cohort definition for asthma as follows: "All patients with ICD-9 493.XX diagnosis codes in their hospital bills." The work group chose this initial definition since 493.XX is the ICD-9 hospital billing code

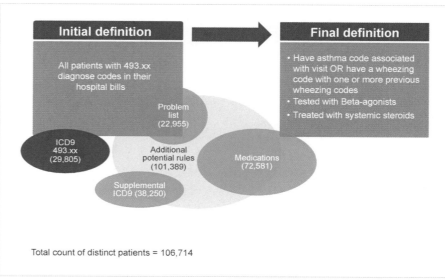

Figure 66: Defining asthma cohort definition
(View Appendix C for larger version)

for asthma cases. Using this initial definition, the work group determined there were about 29,000 patients in the cohort.

The number of patients seemed too low. Some of the clinicians said, "Well, you know we don't always code the condition as asthma. Sometimes we code it as wheezing because we are not sure if it is asthma when the patient initially presents. But many of those cases do turn out to be asthma." The work group involved in the cohort definition and clinical improvement project started to add some supplemental codes that resulted in an additional 38,000 patients. Then they realized that sometimes asthma was noted on the problem list — even though it wasn't coded — so they added those patients as well. Finally, they noted that certain medications were only given to asthma patients (e.g., Albuterol) so they added those patients to the asthma cohort. When all of these rules were considered in the inclusion criteria, 101,000 patients were added to the cohort. Some of the patients overlapped with the original group that was coded as asthma patients, but some were new. As this example shows, having a clinically defined cohort versus just a billing or administratively defined cohort is essential in clinical improvement initiatives.

In this example, the healthcare organization ended up with the following definition for the asthma cohort: patients that have an asthma code associated with a visit or have a wheezing code with one or more previous wheezing codes, and patients that are treated with Beta-agonists or with systemic steroids. After going through this iterative process to build the definition of the cohort, the work group was confident the cohort included all the people with asthma in their patient population.

The Health Catalyst Cohort Builder is an example of a discovery application organizations can use in the process of defining a cohort. In many situations today, when clinicians have questions about patient populations, they have to request data from data analysts who often have a lengthy backlog of requests. Even getting simple queries can take a long time. These questions tend to be iterative resulting in numerous emails between the clinician and the data analyst, which can be a time consuming process. Cohort Builder allows people who are not experts at querying databases to construct complex queries using a simple, self-service interface.

Chapter 6.2 — Evidence-based practice, comparative effectiveness research and levels of evidence

Evidence-based practice (EBP)

Is it taking years — rather than weeks — to put the latest medical evidence into practice? For most organizations, the time between medical knowledge discovery and broad adoption by the majority of clinicians is often measured in years. With patients' health and welfare on the line, everyone agrees these timeframes must change.

A weak clinical content system hinders rapid deployment of new clinical diagnostic and treatment approaches. From a clinical perspective, a clinical content system should consist of standardized knowledge assets, which include evidence-based practice (EBP) guidelines, treatment cascade models, indications for intervention, indications for referral, standing order sets and protocols. The goal of EBP is to systematize how providers decide, for example, when to do surgery and when to order physical therapy.

The most widely used definition of evidence-based practice originated with David Sackett, MD. According to Dr. Sackett, EBP is "the conscientious, explicit and judicious use of current best evidence in making decisions about the care of the individual patient. It means integrating individual clinical expertise with the best available external clinical evidence from systematic research."[91, 92]

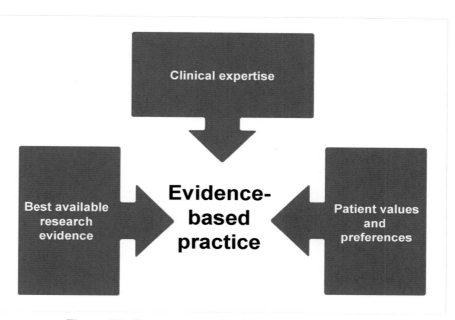

Figure 67: Components of evidence-based practice

EBP is the integration of clinical expertise, patient values and the best research evidence into the decision making process for patient care, as illustrated in Figure 67. Clinical expertise refers to the clinician's accumulated experience, knowledge and clinical skills. The patient brings his or her own personal preferences and unique concerns, expectations and values. The best research evidence generally originates from clinically relevant research that has been conducted using the best available methodology.[93]

Although research is clearly a key element of the care delivery process, clinicians cannot rely solely on the research in their quest to make the best possible decisions for patients. The best decisions result from fully integrating all three key components into the clinical decision-making process — with the goal of optimizing clinical outcomes, addressing patient preferences and achieving the highest possible quality of life and patient satisfaction.

EBP seeks to assess the strength of the evidence as well as the risks and benefits of diagnostic tests and treatments. By using this assessment, clinicians are better able to predict whether a treatment will do more harm than good. Evidence-based medicine seeks to use the experience of a

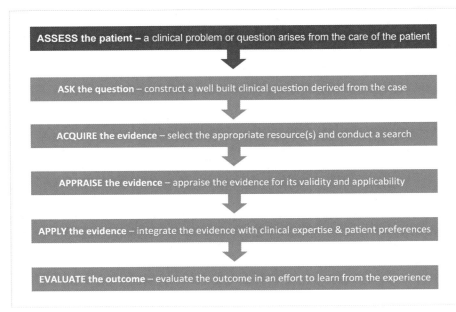

| ASSESS the patient – a clinical problem or question arises from the care of the patient |
| ASK the question – construct a well built clinical question derived from the case |
| ACQUIRE the evidence – select the appropriate resource(s) and conduct a search |
| APPRAISE the evidence – appraise the evidence for its validity and applicability |
| APPLY the evidence – integrate the evidence with clinical expertise & patient preferences |
| EVALUATE the outcome – evaluate the outcome in an effort to learn from the experience |

Figure 68: Steps in the evidence-based process
(View Appendix C for larger version)

population of patients reported in research literature to guide decision-making in routine clinical practice.

As illustrated in Figure 68, EBP is a multi-step process that generally begins with the patient encounter, during which the clinician generates questions about the etiology of the symptoms, the utility of diagnostic tests, the effects of various therapies and the prognosis of the illness or injury. A clinician who promotes and is a good practitioner of EBP must: be knowledgeable and experienced; know how to search the literature for evidence; apply a logical reasoning process to evaluate the validity and applicability of the evidence; and combine the evidence with clinical experience and patient preferences to arrive at the most appropriate decisions. The EBP process also implies the clinician will learn from their experience. If good data is collected as a byproduct of the care delivery process, then the data can be used as part of an ongoing effort to continuously improve patient care in pursuit of better outcomes.

Comparative effectiveness research

The movement toward EBP and the paucity of evidence for many clinical practices has spawned the field of comparative effectiveness research (CER). An Institute of Medicine (IOM) committee has defined comparative effectiveness research as "the generation and synthesis of evidence that compares the benefits and harms of alternative methods to prevent, diagnose, treat and monitor a clinical condition or to improve the delivery of care. The purpose of clinical effectiveness research is to assist consumers, clinicians, purchasers and policy makers to make informed decisions that will improve health care at both the individual and population levels."[94]

An important component of comparative effectiveness research is the concept of pragmatic trials. Clinical trials have been described as either explanatory or pragmatic. Explanatory trials generally measure efficacy — the benefit a treatment produces under ideal conditions, often using carefully defined subjects in a highly controlled care delivery environment. Pragmatic trials measure effectiveness — the benefit the treatment produces in routine clinical practice.

The goal of using an explanatory approach is to further scientific knowledge by recruiting as homogeneous a population as possible. Randomized controlled trials are a form of explanatory trial. By contrast, the design of a pragmatic trial reflects variations between patients that occur in clinical practice and aims to inform treatment choices.[95]

As discussed in chapter 1, Jack Wennberg, MD, and his colleagues at the Dartmouth Institute for Health Policy and Clinical Practice have spent over 40 years documenting the geographic variation in healthcare that patients in the U.S. receive — a phenomenon referred to as practice pattern variation. The Dartmouth researchers concluded: if unwarranted variation were eliminated, the quality of care would increase and healthcare savings of up to 30 percent would be possible — a statistic often repeated in CER.

Several groups have emerged to provide leadership in the area of CER. These include the AHRQ, the IOM and the ECRI Institute. Interested readers can learn more about comparative effectiveness research on their websites. In addition, the IOM has produced an extensive report on comparative effectiveness research.[94]

Understanding levels of evidence

In EBP, it is important to realize that evidence is not the same as proof. The evidence available to clinicians can vary depending on the situation. In some instances, evidence can be so weak it is hardly convincing at all, and in other instances, it can be so strong that no one doubts its correctness. It is therefore important to be able to determine which evidence is the most authoritative. So-called levels of evidence are used for this purpose and specify a hierarchical order for various research designs based on their internal validity.

Internal validity refers to the extent that the results of the underlying research may be biased; it is thus a reference to the degree to which alternative explanations for the outcome are possible. Internal validity is a measure of the strength of the cause-and-effect relationship between an intervention and its outcome. The pure experiment in the form of a randomized controlled trial (RCT) is regarded as the gold standard for documenting internal validity in many disciplines. That is, the study design of RCTs is believed to yield the lowest chance of bias. Non-randomized studies, also referred to as quasi-experimental, observational or correlation studies, are regarded as research designs with lower internal validity. Examples of this type of research design include panel, cohort and case-control studies.

External validity refers to the extent to which the results of a study can be generalized to other situations or populations. Quality improvement trials emphasize external validity, whereas RCTs emphasize internal validity.

The ability to incorporate EBP into clinical care requires a basic understanding of the main research designs underlying the published evidence. Some research designs provide a stronger level of evidence than others based on their inherent characteristics. Systems designed to stratify evidence based on the quality of the evidence have been developed, such as the one developed by the United States Preventive Services Task Force (USPSTF).[96] The USPSTF is an independent panel of experts in primary care and prevention that systematically reviews the evidence of effectiveness and develops recommendations for clinical preventive services. The panel is funded by the U.S. Department of Health and AHRQ.

In creating its recommendations, the USPSTF uses a grading system. The grading system is as follows:

- Grade A: Recommended. There is a high certainty the net benefit is substantial.

- Grade B: Recommended. There is a high certainty the net benefit is moderate, or there is a moderate certainty the net benefit is moderate or substantial.

- Grade C: No recommendation. Clinicians may provide the service to selected patients depending on individual circumstances. However, for most individuals without signs or symptoms there is likely to be only a small benefit.

- Grade D: The task force recommends against this service. There is moderate or high certainty the service has no net benefit or the risk of harm outweighs the benefits.

- Grade I: The current evidence is insufficient to assess the balance of benefits and harms.

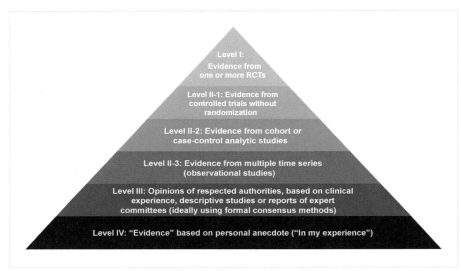

As illustrated in Figure 69, the USPSTF hierarchy of evidence has often been illustrated as a pyramid. The pyramid is an appropriate shape for this graphic, as it represents the quality of research designs by level as well as the quantity of each study design in the body of published literature (i.e., more low quality evidence exists than high quality evidence).

Figure 69: Levels of evidence
(View Appendix C for larger version)

The following is a description of each level of evidence:

● Level I: Evidence from one or more RCTs. A randomized controlled trial is an experimental, prospective study in which participants are randomly allocated into an experimental group or a control group and followed over time for the outcomes of interest. Study participants are randomly assigned to ensure that each participant has an equal chance of being assigned to an experimental or control group, thereby reducing potential bias. Outcomes of interest may be death (mortality), a specific disease state (morbidity) or a numerical measurement, such as blood chemistry level. Randomized controlled trials are frequently used to measure the effectiveness of a particular therapy, especially drug therapies.

A systematic review is a summary of the medical literature that uses explicit methods to perform a comprehensive literature search and critical appraisal of individual randomly controlled trials. These composite studies use appropriate statistical techniques to combine valid studies.[88] Systematic reviews provide the strongest type of evidence, as the authors attempt to find all research on a topic, published and unpublished. The authors then combine the research into a single analysis. Systematic reviews are different than review articles. While systematic reviews are conducted to answer a specific clinical foreground question, review articles provide a broad overview on a topic to answer background questions. Another difference is that the literature search for review articles does not attempt to find all existing knowledge on a topic.

A meta-analysis is a particular type of systematic review that attempts to combine and summarize quantitative data from multiple studies using sophisticated statistical methodologies. Such a strategy strengthens evidence by making the small sample size of individual studies larger, giving the results more statistical power — and therefore, more credibility than the individual studies. Meta-analyses tend not to be comprehensive as only compatible data may be combined into a larger data set.

● Level II-1: Evidence from controlled trials without randomization (quasi-experimental design). Quasi-experimental design is a form of experimental research used extensively in the social sciences and psychology. While many view this approach as unscientific and unreliable, the method has proven useful for measuring social variables. Quasi-experiments resemble quantitative or qualitative experiments, but they lack random allocation of study subjects and proper controls, making good statistical analysis difficult.

- Level II-2: Evidence from cohort or case-control studies. A cohort study is an observational, prospective or retrospective study. A cohort study involves identification of two groups (cohorts) of patients: one that received the exposure of interest, and one that did not. The outcome of interest is measured going forward in time for these cohorts. While at first glance a cohort study may appear similar to a RCT, it differs in one very significant way — the researchers do not assign the exposure or randomize the groups. RCTs are experimental, while cohort studies are observational. Cohort studies may be prospective or retrospective. Retrospective studies involve a major look in the past in an effort to collect information about events that occurred previously. Prospective cohort studies (e.g., the Framingham study) can be extremely time-consuming. It may be necessary to follow a cohort for years or even decades to capture meaningful results. Study participants may no longer be available for follow-up, potentially biasing the results. Retrospective cohort studies, on the other hand, are conducted on data that have already been collected, such as hospital records. A retrospective approach may save time and be less costly.

  A case-control study is an observational, retrospective study, which involves identifying patients who have the outcome of interest (cases) and control patients without the same outcome, and looking back to see if they had the exposure of interest. Because retrospective case-control studies rely on people's memories, they are more prone to error. Also, it may be difficult to measure the exact amount of an exposure in the past.

- Level II-3: Evidence from multiple time series with or without intervention. A case series is a descriptive report on a series of patients with an outcome of interest. No control group is involved. Case series provide the weakest evidence of the study types examined so far, since they describe a relatively small number of patients and no experimental manipulation is involved. Case reports are simply descriptive reports of single patients. Despite their limitations, these study designs can be useful. A case series and case reports often are used to introduce practitioners to unusual and rare conditions, or to point out so-called exceptions to the rule. Dramatic results in uncontrolled trials can be regarded as this type of evidence. Case series and case reports are often the basis for future research using stronger evidence study designs.

- Level III: Evidence based on opinions of respected authorities (ideally using formal consensus methods). As long as one appreciates its limitations, the clinical experience, expertise and judgment of respected healthcare professionals can play an important role in evidence-based medicine. In instances where there is not methodologically sound research to answer a clinical question, expert opinion can be valuable in a clinician's decision-making process, especially when the approach includes agreement among a group of respected authorities using formal consensus methods. In these instances, it becomes extremely important for clinicians to gather baseline data for a process in an effort to assess the outcomes of a process and to determine how the process (and outcome) can be improved over time.

- Level IV: Personal anecdote ("In my experience..."). Although there may be instances where clinicians have little evidence to draw on beyond their individual experience, it should be recognized that this approach is highly prone to bias and often unreliable in producing consistent, best practice outcomes. Unless one's experience is based on some level of evidence, many would argue that this is not evidence at all. In these situations, it becomes extremely important for clinicians to gather baseline data regarding a process in an effort to assess the outcomes of a process, to compare their data with other clinicians involved in the same process of care, and to determine how the process and outcome can be improved over time. At a minimum, clinicians owe it to their patients to gather data in these situations to document outcomes as a part of a continuous improvement and learning process.

The Oxford Centre for Evidence-Based Medicine has developed a more detailed approach for defining levels of evidence. They use a numbering scheme ranging from 1a, homogenous systematic reviews of RCTs, to 5, expert opinion.[97] The Oxford system can be especially useful when comparing articles with similar study designs. Equivalent research designs do not necessarily produce results of equal quality.

Though one would prefer to use research studies high on the pyramid, EBP may need to draw on research designs lower in the evidence hierarchy because of a lack of higher quality published evidence. There are instances where only case reports or bench research may exist on a topic. When making evidence-based decisions in clinical care, clinicians should always strive to select the highest level research design available for the specific clinical situation.

While a double-blinded RCT is the optimum form of evidence, as discussed in chapter 2, a minority of clinical practice is based on RCTs. Thus, clinicians frequently are faced with using lower levels of evidence. Sometimes, the only real evidence they have is their own data. As you move down the pyramid, the need to have control of your own data and to use it wisely in continuous improvement projects increases.

There are numerous definitions for quality improvement. The Rand Corporation has defined quality improvement as "systematic, data-guided activities designed to bring about immediate improvement in the healthcare delivery process."[98] Alternatively, the IOM has defined quality improvement as "a systematic pattern of actions that is constantly optimizing the productivity, communication, and value within an organization in order to achieve the aim of measuring the attributes, properties, and characteristics of a product or service in the context of the expectations and needs of customers and users of that product or service."[20] In contrast, traditional research (RCTs) has been defined as "a systematic investigation including research, development, testing and evaluation designed to develop or contribute to generalizable knowledge."[99]

Quality improvement versus research	
Quality improvement studies	Research studies (RCTs)
Aim: better practice	Aim: new knowledge
Emphasizes external validity	Emphasizes internal validity
Methods:	Methods:
Identify best known practice	Establish clinical equipoise
Open loop (systems-level changes	Closed loop (patient-level changes)
Tests observable (helps spread)	Tests blinded
Stable bias (tolerates "dirty" data)	No bias
Just enough data	All possible data, just in case
Changing hypotheses	Fixed hypotheses
Sequential tests	One large test
Ongoing outcomes tracking	When study ends, data ends

Figure 70: Quality improvement versus research

Not only are traditional research and quality improvement defined differently, but they are governed differently. Quality improvement tends to be governed by entities that focus on quality of care, such as the Joint Commission (TJC), while traditional research is governed by federal regulation and is under Institutional Review Board (IRB) surveillance.

As illustrated in Figure 70, quality improvement studies and traditional research methods (i.e., RCTs) vary in terms of their aims, emphasis and methods. The goal of traditional research is new knowledge, while the goal of quality improvement efforts is better practice. As outlined above, RCTs emphasize internal validity (cause-and-effect relationship), whereas quality improvement research emphasizes external validity (can the result be generalized to other situations or people). Different aims imply different methods. Thus, the methods of the two approaches vary as well.

In reality, there is a synergy between these two approaches. Quality improvement studies can actually enhance traditional research. For example, quality improvement can help determine the external validity (generalizability) of a randomized controlled study's findings. In addition, because one continuously measures in quality improvement studies, the likelihood is actually higher that you will eventually pick up the causality errors you might not find in RCTs.

Chapter 6.3 — Using evidence to identify and eliminate waste

Once the patient cohort is defined, the improvement team is ready to incorporate evidence and start the process of identifying and eliminating waste. While health systems often believe they are unique, in truth they generally are not. The most common clinical and operational problems may be found in all healthcare organizations.

Quality waste relates to process. If a step in a process falls short of expectations or fails, it will often lead to a poor outcome. If one identifies a poor outcome, you either need to fix it or throw it away. Both options cost money. Deming called this re-work. Studies have suggested that quality waste in U.S. hospitals runs between 25 and 40 percent.[100, 101] In 2013, healthcare expenditures in the United States were $2.8 trillion. This means between $700 billion and $1.2 trillion could be recovered and used for other purposes if waste could be eliminated. Some have suggested that U.S. healthcare does not have a cost problem, but rather a waste problem. These staggering numbers would suggest this may be true. The more the U.S. moves towards payment for quality outcomes and not paying for harm (a form of waste), the less tolerable waste will be in healthcare.

If an organization can eliminate waste, their operations costs will go down and their quality will go up — representing a win-win. Modeled on the quality improvement successes that Japan experienced, most organizations outside of healthcare have learned: if they cannot minimize waste, they simply fail. Organizations unable to operate at peak efficiency are not competitive in the market and cannot succeed. They disappear. The elimination of waste has become a condition for entry into most markets.

Historically, healthcare has been rewarded for creating waste. For example, if we caused post-op wound infections, we have been paid to treat it. We have been paid to do unnecessary surgical or other procedures. We have been paid for excess time a patient spent in the ICU on ventilators. However, this is changing. An increasing number of never events (i.e., the kinds of

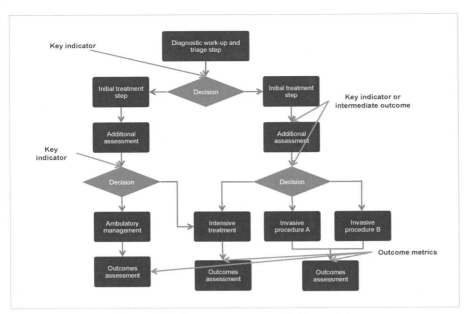

Figure 71: Care process model template
(View Appendix C for larger version)

mistakes that should never have happened) are not reimbursed, payments for specific diagnoses and treatments are being fixed and there is steady downward pressure on reimbursement. All of these trends and others make clinical and operational quality waste increasingly untenable.

As discussed in chapter 5 and illustrated in Figure 71, a care process can be broken down into a set of decisions and activities. Using the evidence-based practice approach discussed in section 6.2, evidence about the best ways to make these decisions or accomplish certain activities may be found in the medical literature. As clinical teams try to understand how their care delivery varies from provider to provider or from one facility to another facility, they can look at how care decisions are currently made and measure the amount of variation existing in the current process compared to the evidence.

For example, the AHRQ has published detailed guidelines that highlight the dangers of inducing labor before a baby is thirty-nine weeks in gestational age.[102] These guidelines were based on a systematic review of 76 research studies originally published between 1964 and 2007.[103] Only under certain specific conditions are the risks of early induction overridden because greater risk to the baby or mother exists. Thus, it is useful to measure what percentage of the time clinicians followed this evidence-based guideline by tracking how many times an induction occurred before thirty-nine weeks without an evidence-based reason. Additionally, clinicians can track how many times a poor outcome, such as an emergency C-section, occurred because the evidence was not followed. This helps the team design tools that match actual care delivery to the evidence.

Using this example, the clinical team might design a knowledge asset like a brochure to educate patients about the risks of early induction. The brochure may reduce the number of mothers asking to be induced before thirty-nine weeks. In addition, the order set for inducing labor could require documentation of the evidence-based reason for inducing early.

Categories of waste

Now let's consider the types of waste commonly seen in healthcare. As shown in Figure 72, there are three common categories of quality waste — ordering waste, workflow waste and defect waste.

Figure 73 illustrates how you can map the Lean types of waste to ordering, workflow or defect waste categories.

Ordering waste

Diagnostic tests can be used to illustrate ordering waste. Figure 74 demonstrates that diagnostic tests can be sorted into three categories: diagnostic, contributory and wasteful. Diagnostic tests aid the physician in making care decisions. Contributory tests may help confirm the diagnosis. Wasteful tests are those that are ordered and do not help in diagnosis or those that are overlooked that would aid diagnosis. Of course, wasteful tests should be eliminated. These tests may be done out of habit, by mistake, based on old evidence or because clinicians are not aware of new evidence. Examples of wasteful tests include duplicate tests, tests that are not helpful in establishing the diagnosis and valid diagnostic tests that do not add any additional information.

Ordering waste

Ordering tests, care, substances and supplies that do not add value

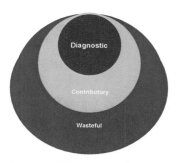

Workflow waste

Variation in efficiency of delivering tests, care and procedures ordered

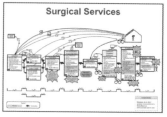

Defect waste

Patient injuries incurred in delivering tests, care and procedures ordered

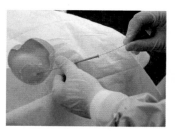

Figure 72: Three forms of waste

Ordering waste	Workflow waste	Defect waste
Over production	Motion	Defects
Inventory	Movement	
Knowledge	Poor processing	
	Waiting	

Figure 73: Categories of waste cross-walked with Lean types of waste

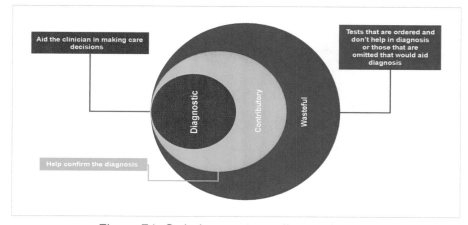

Figure 74: Ordering waste — diagnostic tests
(View Appendix C for larger version)

Let's walk through a heart failure example to illustrate ordering waste (Figure 75). It is not uncommon for patients to be treated for suspected heart failure without confirming the diagnosis. However, without confirming the diagnosis, the treatment may not be appropriate. An echocardiogram is a simple, low cost, noninvasive way to measure the ejection fraction (i.e., the percent of the blood pumped out of the heart ventricle with each stroke). A low ejection fraction is a relatively simple way to confirm heart

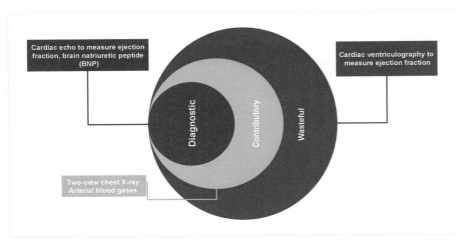

Figure 75: Heart failure ordering waste example
(View Appendix C for larger version)

failure. Brain natriuretic peptide (BNP) is released into the blood when the cardiac muscle is stretched in heart failure. A rising BNP is also diagnostic of heart failure. BNP is another simple, low cost, noninvasive test to confirm the diagnosis of heart failure. Other tests, such as chest X-rays (showing an enlarged heart) and arterial blood gases (showing low oxygen levels), contribute to the diagnosis of heart failure, but they are not unique to heart failure. Given their non-specificity, these tests may be considered wasteful. A cardiac ventriculogram (cardiac catheter used to inject radio opaque dye into the heart) can accurately measure stroke volume (an indirect measure of ejection fraction), but it is expensive and invasive. One would be wiser to try to confirm the diagnosis with less costly and less invasive tests like an echocardiogram or measuring BNP levels. Thus, a cardiac ventriculogram could be considered ordering waste.

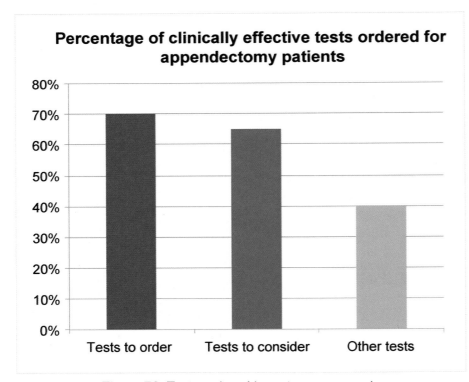

Figure 76: Tests ordered by category example

Another example can be seen in Figure 76, which depicts an analytic application that is evaluating physician habits when writing orders for appendectomy patients. The data reveals that clinically effective tests to order were only ordered, on average, 70 percent of the time. Tests to consider were ordered nearly the same percentage of the time. Other tests were ordered 40 percent of the time. There's a good chance the other tests were wasteful. This analytic application provides the ability to drill down into the data to determine in greater detail what percentage of the time these tests were ordered and under what circumstances. In addition, the order sets that called for specific tests can be viewed. The goal of order sets and workflow modifications should be to make the right thing to do, the easy thing to do.

Workflow waste

Workflow waste differs from ordering waste in that it tends to span departments and often involves inefficiencies in care delivery. Workflow waste occurs either during key value-added steps or in between those steps.

In the chapter on the deployment system, we discussed how to combine Lean with analytics and value stream maps. Value stream maps can help identify workflow waste. By generating knowledge assets such as value stream maps as part of the content system, improvement teams can standardize the value-added steps and eliminate delays.

Figure 77 is an example of a value stream map for an inpatient surgery workflow. The yellow bursts represent waste in the process. The first burst indicates there is tremendous variability in preparing for the surgical cases. The process is nonstandard because each provider has his or her own preference for what to include in the surgical tray. The improvement team could help eliminate this waste by implementing standard surgical preference cards. In this case the intervention would be to standardize the surgeon preference cards.

The other bursts identify an opportunity to standardize the room turnover workflow. The team might create a room turnover checklist that organizes the steps and indicates the typical length of time each step should take. In each of these instances, improvement teams would look to analytics to examine the process and help track adoption of the new standard.

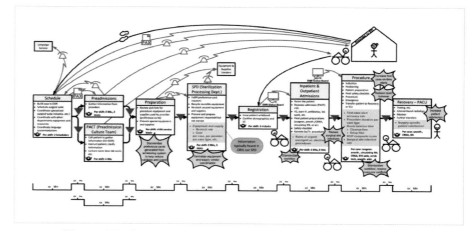

Figure 77: Sample value stream map for inpatient surgery
(View Appendix C for larger version)

Figure 78 demonstrates another operating workflow example. Each bar in the graphic shows the total OR turnover time for the hospital, with the most recent turnover stats shown on the bottom of the graph. The colored segments in each bar represent different stages of the process. For example, the blue segments show the lag between the patient's departure from the OR and the cleanup crew's arrival.

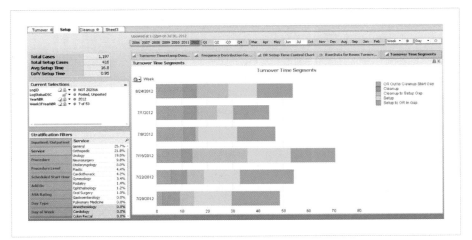

Figure 78: Operating room workflow
(View Appendix C for larger version)

When provided with detailed data about the process, team members are equipped to quickly identify where workflow waste exists and to design counter measures to eliminate the waste. Over time, improvement teams can track whether the counter measures are having the intended impact.

Defect waste

Defect waste represents the third category of waste. Defect waste consists of preventable outcomes that consume additional resources. This includes things like pressure ulcers, transfusion reactions, patient falls and hospital acquired infections.

Most healthcare systems have an incident tracking system, but incident tracking only accounts for incidents that are severe enough for the clinician to fill out an incident report. Incident tracking does not capture all the near misses or instances that are almost bad enough to be tracked.

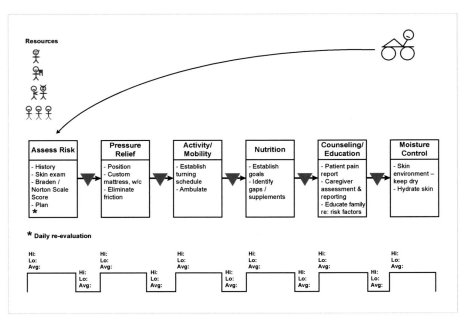

Figure 79: Pressure injury prevention
(View Appendix C for larger version)

Figure 79 shows a pressure injury example. Any patient who is going to be admitted to a certain unit of the hospital for more than a couple hours should be assessed for risk of a pressure injury. For patients deemed at risk, various pressure relief interventions should be used: a special mattress, specific activities, nutrition, etc. As long as clinicians check 100 percent of patients, they can make sure the patients who need special provisions receive them and that other patients do not. Clinicians can use an analytic application to examine historical trends to help inform them of the types of workflow changes or knowledge assets that may need to be implemented. Then they apply the principles of the content system to create several tools to reduce the incidence of pressure ulcers.

It is very important that waste reduction be systematic, not limited to a specific department and that a consistent approach be used across clinical programs. As shown in Figure 80, to accomplish this improvement teams should keep strengthening the three systems and revisiting important questions.

Strong analytics are used to uncover and provide information on the three kinds of waste. The data is unlocked, data gathering is automated and the data is used to reveal the highest priorities and define the necessary cohorts of patients. This can be used to build dashboards with actionable metrics that allow an organization to change behaviors.

	Ordering	Workflow	Defect
Analytic system	Are we following clinical effectiveness guidelines?	Are we delivering the care efficiently?	Are we delivering the care safely?
Deployment system	Clinical program	Clinical support service	Clinical support service
Content system	What should be done?	How can it be done efficiently?	How can it be done safely?

Figure 80: Sample questions to improve your 3 systems

Strong deployment is used to implement and sustain less wasteful practices. Permanent teams integrating clinicians and technical experts are established. These teams will engage in Agile, iterative work processes involving high levels of communication. Lean principles are combined with analytics so improvement teams can uncover root causes and sustain gains.

Finally, strong content is used to hone and improve clinical practices. Advanced medical knowledge within your organization or knowledge that is discovered in another organization is used to establish a new standard within weeks, instead of years. Going forward, these practices should be continually improved upon. In combination, all three of these systems — analytic, deployment and content — can ignite change.

The categories of waste described above relate to the treatment of individual patients. There is another type of waste that relates to populations and societies as a whole.

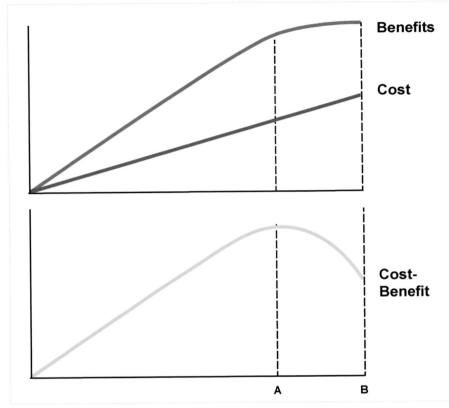

Figure 81: Useful additions to care

In chapter 2, we discussed Donabedian's concept of the maximalist and optimalist approach illustrated in Figure 81.

Instead of thinking of the care of one patient at a time, imagine that you are tasked with care delivery to a population and you have a finite (limited) number of resources. Given the direction of healthcare economics, this is not a stretch. In fact, this reality is currently unfolding in healthcare. Because of many competing demands, it is unlikely that more money will be allocated to clinical care delivery. We have to spend the resources we are currently given in a better, more efficient manner.

In such a situation, you are likely going to want to pay attention to the cost-benefit curve. This is the slope of the green line divided by the slope of the red line in the Figure 81. Donabedian pointed out that if you want maximum benefit across a population you want to be at the peak of the "cost-benefit" curve (point A on the lower yellow graph). Donabedian called this an optimalist approach because an optimalist seeks maximum benefit across a population. If you are going to spend more treatment money, you would prefer to find a patient located before point A where the slope of the curve is still going up, indicating the patient will get more benefit than a patient beyond point A. The difference is focusing on the whole (i.e., the population) rather than solely on an individual patient.

Donabedian's whole purpose was to talk about the ethics of patient care from a different perspective (i.e., the population as opposed to an individual patient). If you are talking about a population, you have a responsibility to ask patients as a group how much healthcare they want to buy, at what cost and what benefit.

Donabedian argued this was not a decision for clinicians to make. Instead, it was the decision of the population of patients (i.e., society). The obligation of clinicians in this circumstance is to help society understand the trade-offs. We have a professional responsibility to do this. Ethically, it is our responsibility to inform society. It is society's ethical responsibility to decide how much to spend and where to spend it.

It is unethical to tolerate any kind of waste in healthcare delivery. As a caring clinician, executive or administrator, we have a professional responsibility to think not only about the patient in front of us, but all patients. It is becoming increasingly clear that resources are finite. Every time we waste resources on one patient, we deny resources to other patients. As respected professionals, we have an ethical responsibility to think of all patients. It is important that clinicians and administrators see this need and get out in front of it. Nature abhors a vacuum. If we do not deal with this reality, someone else will and that would not necessarily be a good thing from society's perspective. At a minimum, we need to play a participatory leadership role because we have the expertise and knowledge to do so. This is a tough standard, and it is not easy, but it is a role we must play. This is what the pioneers like Sir William Osler were willing to do over a century ago. They provided this type of leadership. It is now time for clinical and operational leaders in our generation to do the same. We are living on borrowed time. Healthcare is approaching the zero hour.

Chapter 6.4 — Standardizing care delivery through practice protocols and shared baselines

Next, we need to turn our attention to the steps a healthcare organization can take to establish a standard process using shared baselines that are reflected in practice protocols. As an initial step, let's discuss the role of practice protocols in evidence-based medicine.

The role of practice protocols in evidence-based medicine

As healthcare transforms, the traditional craft of medicine is being supplanted with a more profession-based approach for the reasons outlined in chapter 3. The idea that every physician, nurse or administrator is a personal expert, relying solely on his or her personal commitment to excellence is no longer acceptable. We are moving from medicine practice as individual heroism to medicine as a team sport.

David Eddy, MD, was the first to suggest that the core assumption of the craft of medicine is untenable.[104] Under the craft of medicine, the idea was that when a physician faced a patient, by some fundamentally human process called the art of medicine or clinical judgment, the physician would synthesize all of the important information about the patient, relevant research and experiences with previous patients to determine the best course of action.

Over the last thirty years, however, it has become apparent that the published evidence for most of what we do in clinical care is limited. Over the same period of time, clinical care has become increasingly and overwhelmingly complex. As illustrated in Figure 82, these trends coupled with widespread variations in beliefs and human limitations in the face of complexity has led to well documented clinical uncertainty, massive variation in care and unacceptable levels of inappropriate care.

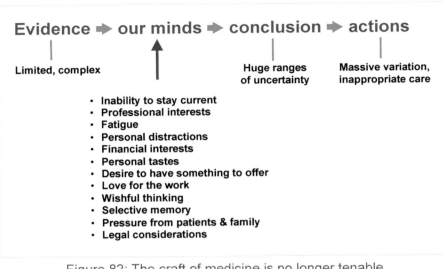

Figure 82: The craft of medicine is no longer tenable

The movement toward evidence-based medicine has led to a growing acceptance of practice protocols in clinical care. Practice protocols are an important part of a profession-based practice. They support an environment of professional accountability where groups of physicians and other professionals manage similar patients in similar settings, discuss best patient care practices, inform their decisions based on the medical literature and expert opinion, and use credible data to assess their performance and outcomes.

Developing a shared common baseline

Every health system and hospital needs a more systematic approach to learning about evidence, to get the evidence integrated quickly and efficiently into the normal work processes, and to avoid the "if it wasn't invented here, we have to reinvent it" mentality. Sometimes physicians will call this cookie-cutter medicine. However, for the simple or common standard clinical cases, all clinicians should want to provide care in a standard way because it allows for the creation of shared common baselines and supports improvement efforts. This allows well-trained clinicians to focus on the more complex cases that are the roughly 20 percent of outlier cases where their judgment and expertise are most important. For the more simple cases, standardized processes work just fine.

In creating a practice protocol, clinicians select a high priority care process, generate an evidence-based best practice guideline and appropriately blend the guideline into the flow of clinical work (e.g., staffing, supplies, physical layout, information flow, and training) as illustrated in Figure 83.

The first step to evidence integration is to select a high-priority care process that has high variation as defined by analytical tools like Health Catalyst's Key Process Analysis application — the tool that was illustrated in chapter 4.

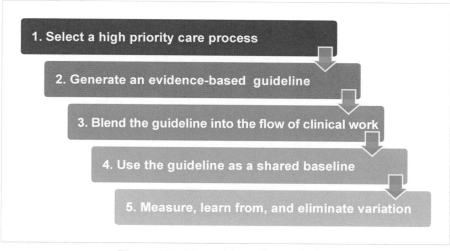

1. Select a high priority care process
2. Generate an evidence-based guideline
3. Blend the guideline into the flow of clinical work
4. Use the guideline as a shared baseline
5. Measure, learn from, and eliminate variation

Figure 83: Shared baseline solution

From there, an improvement team can generate an evidence-based guideline and blend it into the workflow. This could involve standardizing diagnostic algorithms, order sets, intervention criteria, supplies, department layouts, and patient and provider education materials. The improvement team will also design the best way to measure utilization of the guideline.

Then, they will use the guideline as part of a standard protocol using a shared baseline. A shared common baseline requires that a protocol be standard. That is, all care providers involved in any given care process must use a standard protocol. Without using a standard protocol, it is impossible to develop a meaningful shared common baseline. A shared common baseline is essential in defining baseline performance for a care process and in allowing care providers to know if future enhancements to a process represent an improvement.

In a standard protocol-based care environment, clinicians can vary care based on individual patient needs and desires. Once again, this is a key element of Lean production — so-called mass customization. That is, front-line clinicians are able to address complexity and drive out waste using standardized processes while also providing room to adapt to individual customer needs. This allows caregivers to focus on a relatively narrow band defined by a patient's individuality where their expertise and experience really make a difference. The protocol standardizes the mundane work so that it happens automatically, using a measurement system to assure it is happening consistently and correctly, while allowing the caregiver to use their intellect where it is needed most — the roughly 20 percent of care that needs to be modified to match the needs or characteristics of an individual patient. When clinicians do vary from a standard protocol, the reason for varying should be captured, so everyone can learn from it.

Once a protocol is implemented, clinicians can measure outcomes and learn from their experience. Teams of clinicians involved in a given care process can manage cycles of measurement and learning, repeating the process until variation is eliminated. Specifically, improvement teams want to eliminate variation caused by different healthcare professionals yet retain variation arising from different patient conditions.

Evidence-based protocols and shared baselines actually make care easier. When properly integrated into workflow, protocols have been shown to help physicians become substantially more productive. With good protocols in place, physicians do not need to worry about details that do not require their intellect. Those details happen automatically. The standardized protocol assures these details get done reliably every time. This yields more time for clinicians to see patients and generate additional value for patients. However, it is important to remember protocols need to be continuously improved as new published evidence becomes available and as care teams learn more about the care they deliver.

Protocols can also be a very effective training tool (as they have been for a long time) — think of the Washington Manual that medical students and residents have used for decades. It is filled with standard protocols. These published tools had at least one drawback — they lacked a shared common baseline to determine how well you were doing and the ability to thoughtfully measure as you implemented changes to see if they were making a difference. A well designed EHR and enterprise data warehouse (EDW) creates the ability to collect the data you need to understand and improve protocols over time.

A growing body of evidence suggests that a profession-based practice using standard protocols has many advantages. It produces better outcomes for patients. It eliminates waste, reduces costs and increases available resources for patient care. It puts caring professionals back in control of care delivery where they belong. It is the foundation for useful shared electronic data.

Chapter 6.5 — Tools to help accelerate waste identification and elimination

Now that we have learned how to define clinically driven cohorts, how to use evidence to identify and eliminate waste and how to standardize care delivery through shared common baselines, let's consider what tools are necessary to accelerate waste identification and elimination.

When an organization or a nation tries to implement value on a broad scale (i.e., safe, high-quality care, at the lowest possible cost), it requires ready access to good data. This, in turn, requires the broad implementation of EHRs. It also requires you to think of an EHR in terms of its ability to build care management capability. The EHR needs to be a foundation for building and supporting care management. It is also necessary to collect the data required to determine shared common baselines and to document improvement as processes are improved over time.

Just as in the case of protocols, standardization is important when implementing an EHR. When you tailor any enterprise information technology system (e.g., EHR, finance, human resources, patient satisfaction, etc.), an organization can lose its advantages if a non-standard approach is taken with the system — especially when it is time to upgrade to a new version of the system with new capabilities.

If the EHR has been heavily customized, it will cost the organization more and be more difficult to implement the new version of the system. In addition, if data is entered in an EHR in a non-standard manner, it impacts data integrity in the EDW.

Healthcare organizations need an EDW and other elements of an effective analytical platform that supports selective information tracking required for mass customization. Using one

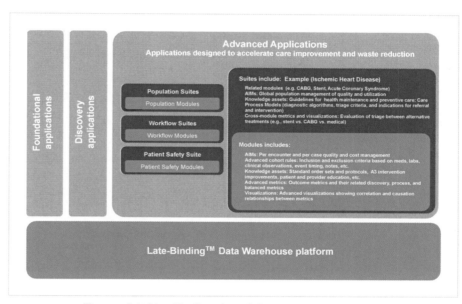

Figure 84: Health Catalyst Advanced Applications
(View Appendix C for larger version)

healthcare analytic vendor as an example, Health Catalyst offers three suites of tools, and each suite supports identifying and eliminating waste in each of the three categories: ordering, workflow and defects. These tools are shown in Figure 84.

Population suites help improvement teams manage clinical processes and determine the types of care being ordered. Workflow suites help manage the efficiency of care delivery within departments. Patient safety suites support the safe delivery of care. Within the application suites, clinical work process modules exist. For example, a population suite for ischemic heart disease would have modules for each of the clinical work processes within that care process family, such as open-heart surgery, stents and angina.

As reviewed in chapter 3, a process is a series of actions or steps that are taken in order to achieve a particular goal or outcome. A system is generally made up of a collection of interlinked processes that collectively allow an organization to achieve its goals on behalf of customers. Process modeling is an activity whereby those who understand a process create a representation of the process using a variety of graphical tools. The goal of process modeling is generally to create a reasonable representation of a given process in an effort to eliminate unnecessary steps (waste) and optimize specific desired outcomes.

In order to understand any clinical process, care providers need to use the basic process improvement and team tools used in any other industry. These tools are simple and easy to use. They are used to help describe and organize a process, and to focus process improvement efforts. The most commonly used process improvement tools are:

- Flow (conceptual flow, decision flow) charts
- Value stream mapping
- Cause and effect (Ishikawa, fishbone) diagrams
- Tally sheets
- Pareto charts
- Statistical process control (SPC) and statistical process control charts

Flow charts

Flow charts are easy-to-understand diagrams showing how steps in a process fit together. This makes them useful tools for communicating how processes work, and for clearly documenting how a particular job is done and how a particular outcome is achieved. The act of mapping a process out in flow chart format helps teams clarify their understanding of a given process and helps them think about where the process can be streamlined or improved.

A flow chart can be used to:

- Define and analyze processes
- Build a step-by-step picture of the process for analysis, discussion and communication
- Define, standardize or identify areas for improvement in a process

By conveying the information about a process in a step-by-step flow chart, teams can then concentrate more intently on each individual step in the process as well as the overall process.

The types of flow charts and the types of symbols used in flow charts are summarized in Figure 85.

The following graphics demonstrate two examples of flow charts from healthcare improvement projects — Figure 86 depicts the discharge process from a rehab unit and Figure 87 illustrates an adverse drug event (ADE) detection process.

Value stream mapping

Value stream mapping is a Lean tool that employs a flow diagram documenting in high detail every step of a process. Many Lean practitioners see value stream mapping as the fundamental tool to identify waste, reduce process cycle times and implement process improvement. A value stream map is often the key tool used in Lean improvement efforts.

Value stream mapping can help improvement teams map, visualize, understand the flow of patients, materials, information and decisions in a process. The "value stream" is all of the actions required to complete a particular process. The goal of value steam mapping is to identify improvements that can be made to reduce waste (e.g., patient wait times), improve cycle times (e.g., OR room turn around) and identify and implement process improvements.

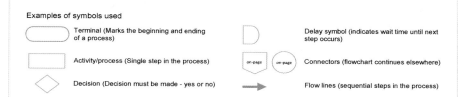

Types of flow charts:

- **Work-flow** – physical flow of people, work, documents, information
- **Deployment** – flow of work processes and individual responsibilities (matrix diagram)
- **Outline** – describes principal features of a process
- **Top-down,** hierarchical – helps show systems
- **Detailed** – most time consuming (industrial model)

Examples of symbols used

Terminal (Marks the beginning and ending of a process)

Activity/process (Single step in the process)

Decision (Decision must be made - yes or no)

Delay symbol (indicates wait time until next step occurs)

Connectors (flowchart continues elsewhere)

Flow lines (sequential steps in the process)

Figure 85: Types of flow charts and flow chart symbols
(View Appendix C for larger version)

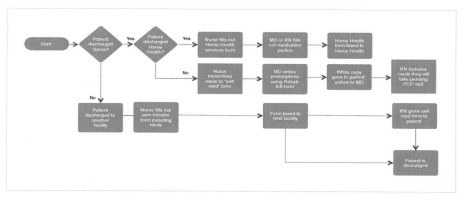

Figure 86: Rehab discharge process
(View Appendix C for larger version)

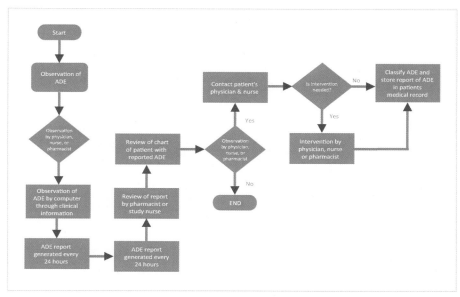

Figure 87: Detection of adverse drug events process
(View Appendix C for larger version)

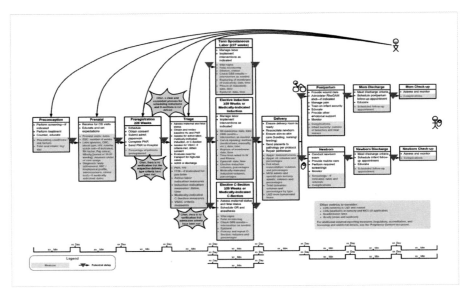

Figure 88: Sample pregnancy value stream map
(View Appendix C for larger version)

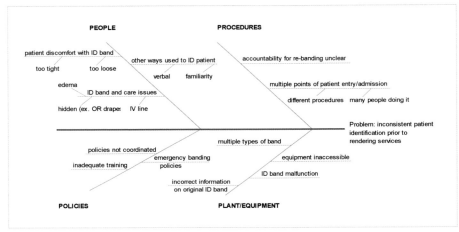

Figure 89: Sample patient identification fishbone diagram
(View Appendix C for larger version)

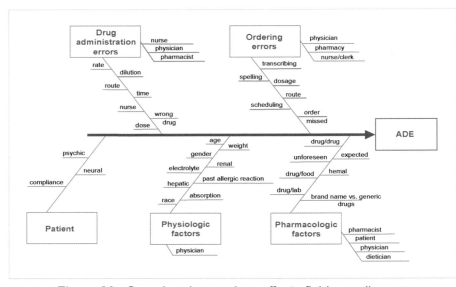

Figure 90: Sample adverse drug effects fishbone diagram
(View Appendix C for larger version)

To accurately map a process, it is important to obtain high-quality, reliable data about the flow of information and the time spent at (or between) steps. Accurately timing process steps and using multi-departmental teams is essential to obtain a true picture of what's going on in any process.

An example of a value stream map was shown in the workflow waste discussion (Figure 77). Another example is shown in Figure 88.

Cause and effect (Ishikawa, fishbone) diagrams

Once a high level process has been mapped, a performance improvement team often needs to discuss the potential causes of a defect in one or more of the process steps. A cause and effect (Ishikawa, fishbone) diagram has traditionally been used to highlight potential causes.

A cause and effect diagram is a graphical tool that enables the visualization of causal relationships between variables in a process. The so-called fishbone diagram can be used to structure a brainstorming session by sorting inputs or causes into useful categories — two examples are shown in Figures 89 and 90. Causes are typically arranged according to their level of importance or detail, resulting in a depiction of relationships and a hierarchy of events. The diagram can help search for root causes, identify areas where there may be problems, compare the relative importance of different causes, uncover bottlenecks in a process, identify why a process is not working and discover areas for improvement.

Talley sheets

The tally sheet is a simple and effective tool that is often useful in quality improvement projects. It is a convenient tool for both qualitative and quantitative data gathering and analysis. It is commonly used to collect data on quality problems and to determine the frequency of events. It is a good first step in understanding the nature of the problem as it provides a uniform data collection tool. The tally sheet can be very useful to help distinguish opinions from facts.

Using a tally sheet is appropriate when the data can be observed and collected repeatedly by either the same person or in the same location. It is also an effective tool when collecting data on frequency and identifying patterns of events, problems, defects, and defect location and for identifying defect causes.

For example, the tally sheet is useful for understanding the reasons patients are arriving late for appointments, causes for delays in getting the lab results back, etc. It is also useful in determining frequency of occurrence, such as number of people in line for blood tests at 6:00 a.m., 6:15 a.m., etc., to understand staffing needs. Tally sheets can also be useful in clinical quality improvement projects. Figure 91 is an example of a simple tally sheet used in a laboratory improvement project.

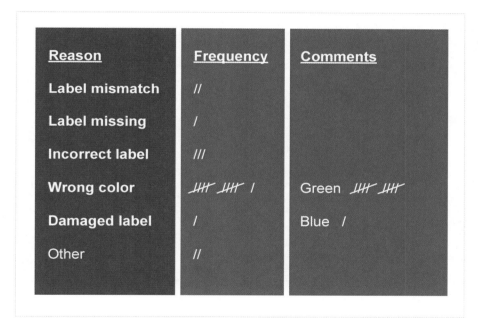

Figure 91: Tally sheet example

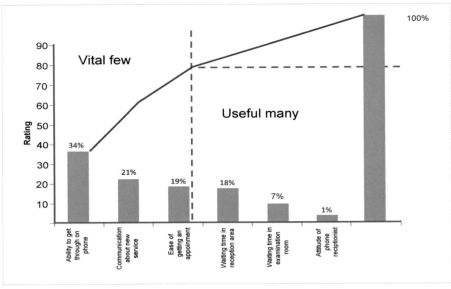

Figure 92: Pareto analysis — family practice patient survey
(View Appendix C for larger version)

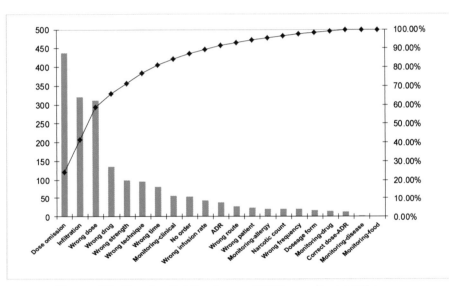

Figure 93: Pareto distribution — 2007 reported ADE types
(View Appendix C for larger version)

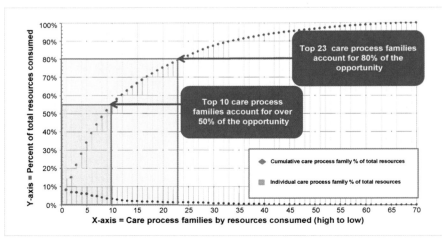

Figure 94: Key Process Analysis
(View Appendix C for larger version)

Pareto charts

The Pareto principle was discussed in chapter 4. The value of the Pareto principle is that it reminds you to focus on the most important causes of poor quality in a process — the so-called vital few — as opposed to the less important causes — the useful many, as portrayed in Figure 92.

The Pareto distribution is a probability distribution that is used in the description of many observable phenomena. An example of a typical healthcare Pareto distribution is illustrated in Figure 93. It shows the causes of ADEs at a regional medical center. The top five causes of adverse drug events produce 80 percent of the ADEs reported at this medical center.

The Pareto principle also applies to the resources consumed by care processes. That is, the top 20 percent of care processes typically consume 80 percent of resources making them a key target for improvement efforts, as shown in Figure 94.

Statistical process control (SPC) charts

Improvement occurs over time. Therefore, determining if improvement has actually happened and if it is lasting requires observing results over time. Run charts are graphs of data over time. They represent one of the most important quality improvement tools for assessing the effectiveness of a change.

As discussed in chapter 4, statistical process control (SPC) is a quality improvement method, which is applied in order to monitor and control a process. Monitoring and controlling the process can help ensure a process operates at its full potential, thus achieving the best possible outcomes with a minimum (if not an elimination) of waste. Statistical process control can generally be applied to any process where the output can be measured. Control charts are the primary method of displaying statistical process control results.

The derivation and use of statistical process control and statistical process control charts in quality improvement was discussed in considerable detail in chapter 4.3. The reader is referred to that chapter for further information regarding statistical process control charts.

The Institute for Health (IHI) model for improvement

IHI recommends the use of the IOM Model for Improvement as a framework to guide improvement work. The Model for Improvement is a simple, yet effective tool for accelerating improvement. Illustrated in Figure 95, the model uses a Plan-Do-Study-Act (PDSA) cycle.

The PDSA cycle can be repeated many times in the continuous improvement process, as shown in Figure 96.

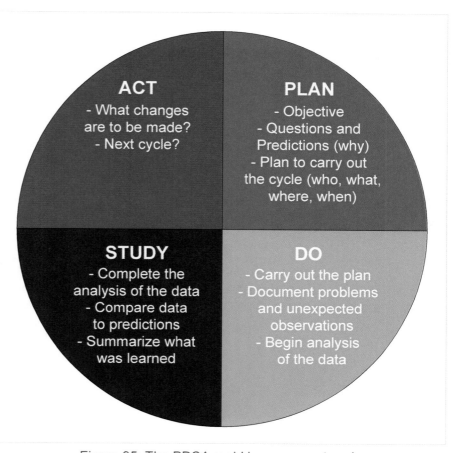

Figure 95: The PDSA rapid improvement cycle

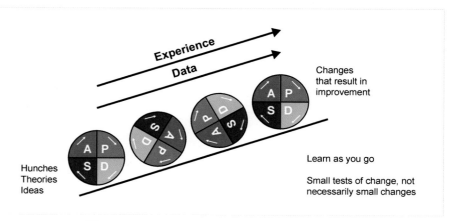

Figure 96: Repeated use of the PDSA cycle

The IHI Model for Improvement involves several logical steps, including forming the right improvement team, setting aims, establishing measurable goals, selecting and testing changes (improvements) for a process, implementing changes and spreading improvements. The reader is encouraged to review the IHI's recommendations in detail.[92]

An example of applying quality improvement methods to healthcare: Intermountain Healthcare

Under the visionary leadership of Brent James, MD, and David Burton, MD, Intermountain Healthcare has a well-deserved reputation as a world leader in the application of quality improvement concepts and methods in pursuit of clinical and operational excellence. As a result of their focus on quality improvement, Intermountain Healthcare hospitals and clinics are routinely recognized as among the best in the country in terms of their quality, safety and cost outcomes.

Intermountain Healthcare has invested extensively in programs to educate and engage their clinical and operational leaders in continuous quality improvement. These investments in people have proven to be remarkably successful. As a part of the educational programs, each course participant is required to do an improvement project in order to graduate. The purpose of the project is to provide hands-on experience in quality improvement, to produce real results and to provide a practical way to learn what works. As a guide, Dr. James has students/ teams use Juran's model of the Diagnostic Journey, the Remedial Journey and Holding the Gains, as shown in Figure 97.

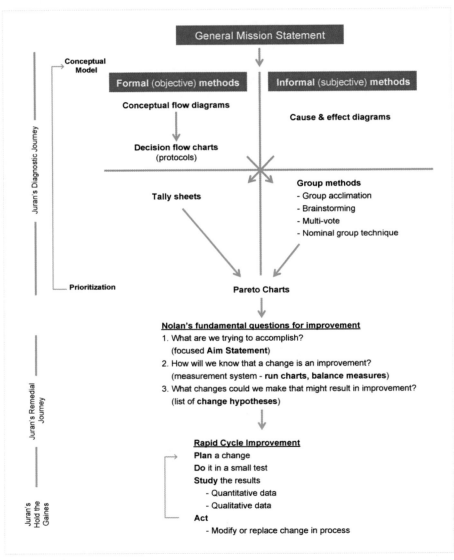

Figure 97: Modeling processes
(View Appendix C for larger version)

The Juran Diagnostic Journey goes from the initial analysis of the evidence (symptoms) of the quality problem and ends with the determination of the cause or causes of the problem. The journey includes activities common to all improvement projects.

- Analyze the evidence (symptoms) of the quality problem

- Formulate theories regarding the cause or causes of the problem

- Test the theories

During this stage of the quality improvement journey, teams have a variety of tools at their disposal, including conceptual diagrams, decision flow diagrams, cause and effect diagrams, tally sheets, group methods and Pareto charts. By taking a logical and informed approach using these tools, the quality improvement team will eventually establish the real cause or causes of the quality problem or defect. At that point, the diagnostic journey is over, and the remedial journey begins.

The Juran Remedial Journey begins with the identified known cause or causes for a quality problem or defect and ends with an effective remedy in place. The activities of the project team at this stage include:

- Identify alternative solutions

- Take action to remedy the problem

- Deal with any resistance to change

- Establish controls to hold the gains

A key step in both the IHI Model for Improvement and the Intermountain Healthcare approach is the development of an effective Aim Statement. Aim Statements are specific, measurable, time sensitive, written statements of what a quality improvement team will be focusing on as they strive to improve a process. A good Aim Statement will help keep an improvement project focused and on course.

In general, an Aim Statement should include a few key elements that seek to answer three questions (adapted from The Foundation for Improvement by Thomas W. Nolan, et al.):

1. What is the improvement team trying to accomplish?

2. Who is the specific target population?

3. What changes can we make that will result in an improvement?

The aim should be as concise as possible and be outcomes focused. It is not uncommon for a team to test and refine an Aim Statement in an effort to make it as concise and focused as possible.

A good Aim Statement sets stretch goals. Whether an improvement team hits the goal is less important than whether they advance learning and improve outcomes. The team should measure performance by how much they improve care, not whether they hit any given stretch goal. If the team fails, it should fail in the direction of improvement.

Once the Aim Statement is in place, the identified solutions are implemented and refined as a part of a rapid cycle improvement process using one or more PDSA cycles. In applying the remedy, it is important to recognize that this often means change and change can result in resistance. Thus, the Juran model stresses the importance of dealing with the resistance to change.

See chapter 5 for examples of Aim Statements.

In conclusion

At this point, we have discussed in detail the three systems care delivery organizations need to adopt in order to excel. Organizations need a strong analytic system to standardize measurement work, a strong deployment system to standardize organizational work and a strong content system to standardize knowledge work. Together, these three systems can help an organization improve clinical effectiveness, reduce waste and ensure patient safety.

What happens if an organization strengthens only one of its three systems? If an organization focuses only on analytics, they become information system centric. They end up strengthening the information request queue without ever putting the data to work. If deployment is the main focus, an organization becomes organization centric. Clinicians stop attending meetings because solid evidence and actionable measures are lacking. And if content takes the front seat, an organization finds itself in a research centric model with great academic ideas, but no data to support them and no one willing to deploy.

If even one of the systems is weak, an organization is left with an incomplete plan. Without analytics, an organization can become Lean centric. Quick improvements are made but you will have trouble measuring them as the projects pile up and the improvements are not sustained. Without deployment, an organization ends up with a lot of small, isolated science projects that never get rolled out across facilities. And without content, an organization has what could be referred to as paved cow paths. You have automated — and solidified — processes that have not been refined.

Only by strengthening all three systems can you deliver evidence-based care and drive scalable, sustainable improvements in cost and quality. It is in the confluence of these three systems that enables an organization to ignite change.

As one implements change in the clinical realm, it is important to emphasize once again that care providers are motivated by their professional values. The vast majority of clinicians are aligned by their shared professional values. Most clinicians want to do the best thing for the patients they serve and they have a strong desire to be the best they can be in that service. While money is important, it is also important to align improvement efforts with professional values. Tapping this innate desire of clinicians to be the best they can be is a key element of success in continuous improvement. It can be key to overcoming cultural resistance to change in clinical care. And, it is fundamentally important to transform healthcare.

We will now turn our attention in part three to see what success looks like for organizations that successfully apply the concepts, tools and methods reviewed in this section, as well as the future of healthcare analytics and associated technologies.

PART THREE: LOOKING INTO THE FUTURE

Introduction

Once an organization has successfully implemented the three systems framework, it will have established the foundation for a new, more engaging and more powerful way of delivering care. This foundation will enable organizations to deal with the challenges currently facing healthcare. In part 3, we will look into the future from two perspectives. With respect to the near term, chapter 7 will provide real world examples of successful clinical and operational improvement initiatives from organizations that have implemented the three systems framework. In chapter 8, we will look a little further into the future at impending innovations related to population management, care delivery system design and technology-enabled care model redesign, and the impact these innovations will likely have on the future of healthcare analytics.

7 REAL WORLD EXAMPLES PROVIDE A GLIMPSE INTO OUR FUTURE

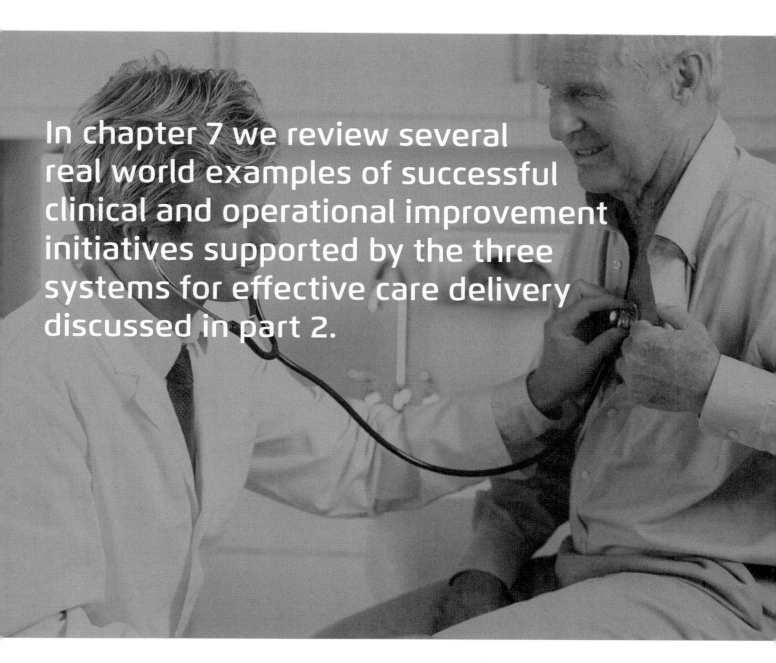

In chapter 7 we review several real world examples of successful clinical and operational improvement initiatives supported by the three systems for effective care delivery discussed in part 2.

Now that we have reviewed the systems, methods and tools required to effectively address the quality, safety, waste and cost challenges confronting healthcare, it is time to look at the end game. What will success look like? It is not necessary to imagine what success will look like. We can actually look at real world examples.

A growing number of clinicians are finding that by working together to analyze evidence-based practices and selecting the most effective practices they are enhancing their sense of professional satisfaction, improving patients' experiences and delivering better patient outcomes. Continuous improvement can be rewarding and fun, and it is certainly in line with our professional values. It requires data and a willingness to honestly seek and use evidence-based practices. When you get together with other clinicians you can agree on what quality is and start measuring your performance. You can share and debate the data and identify practices that are effective and efficient. In the process, everyone learns. This is continuous improvement.

> " Process improvement is not just a nice idea. Increasingly, groups of innovative clinicians are forming, identifying best practices, measuring outcomes and continuously improving care for the patients they serve ... "

Process improvement is not just a nice idea. Increasingly, groups of innovative clinicians are forming, identifying best practices, measuring outcomes and continuously improving care for the patients they serve in healthcare organization across our country. Disease by disease, they are attacking the illness burden that inflicts humanity, and in the process they are improving the value of care being delivered to patients.

This can be an exciting and energizing experience for clinicians involved in improvement because the reform debate has suddenly shifted to what matters most to you and your patients — the value of care your patients receive. The future mandates that healthcare organizations embrace the Institute for Healthcare Improvement (IHI) triple AIM: better care for individuals, better health for populations and cost management. Let's look at some examples of clinicians and healthcare organizations that are achieving operational and clinical process improvement success.

Rapid cycle clinical process improvement

Background

Texas Children's Hospital in Houston, Texas, is one of the premier children's hospitals in the United States. In an industry shifting to value-based care delivery models, Texas Children's is focusing on quality improvement, data management and its ability to manage high-risk patient populations.

Texas Children's leaders had long been convinced that technology could play a key role in improving the quality and coordination of care among its patient population. Hoping it would transform raw clinical and financial data into meaningful information that the hospital could use to guide its delivery of care and services, they began implementation of an enterprise-wide electronic health record (EHR) in 2008.

The EHR proved tremendously valuable as the means of digitizing care across the hospital. However, despite implementing an EHR, Texas Children's — like many healthcare organizations — struggled with cumbersome processes for analyzing populations, defining patient cohorts and implementing improvement programs that drove measurable and sustainable improvement. In reality, the newly digitized EHR data was hard to extract and combine with other data sources in a timely fashion. TCH found that it took between three and six months for analysts to deliver clear answers to key clinical and operational questions using EHR data. As a result, executives and clinicians were not able to effectively leverage the data to make timely, data-driven, financially sustainable improvements in care for either individuals or specific populations. As Myra Davis, senior vice president and CIO described the situation, "Our clinicians thought the EHR was a silver bullet to get the data they needed," she said. "The comments I would hear were, 'I can't get the right data,' or 'The IT staff doesn't understand what I need from the records.' It created nothing but frustration."

> "Our clinicians thought that the EHR would be a silver bullet to get the data they needed for quality improvement and operational reporting and they blamed IT when the information wasn't forthcoming
>
> -Myra Davis, senior vice president and CIO

Texas Children's learned that while implementing an EHR is clearly a necessary step toward data-driven delivery of care, the EHR alone is not enough without an enterprise data warehouse (EDW) that enables an enterprise-wide, consistent view of data from many sources.

After realizing that the EHR was not the silver bullet that had been expected, Texas Children's leaders decided to take a bold, integrated approach to healthcare analytics, data management and quality improvement. Beginning in September 2011, the hospital worked with Health Catalyst to implement an analytic, deployment and content framework for value-based transformation.

As the first step, the framework introduces an EDW to improve measurement and analytics throughout the organization. The flexible and adaptable Late-Binding™ Data Warehouse platform is designed to handle the massive quantities of data in large healthcare organizations. The EDW organized Texas Children's data into a single source of truth that serves as a foundation for data-driven improvement. This technology enabled Texas Children's to eliminate the manual data-gathering process and automate data distribution.

The EDW technology provided a necessary foundation. But Texas Children's leaders also understood that technology alone would not enable them to improve the overall value of care. Doing that would also require a fundamental culture change — a culture focused on data-driven continuous improvement. So Texas Children's implemented two additional aspects of the framework:

> Permanent, integrated workgroup teams that identify areas for care improvement and building evidence-based practices into the care delivery workflow.

> Advanced healthcare analytics applications that run on the EDW platform to prioritize, track and interpret iterative improvement.

Texas Children's moved forward to put a three system framework for effective care delivery (analytic, deployment and content) into action, beginning with implementing the EDW. Implementation was completed in just three months — a phenomenally fast time. By rolling out a more flexible and adaptable analytic system, Texas Children's overcame significant data barriers to process improvement and has embraced a data-driven methodology for rapid-cycle process improvement.

> "Additionally, Texas Christian's established a formal entity, the Evidence Based Outcomes Center (EBOC) that spearheads the organization's efforts to effectively use data to improve care and to make clinical practice consistent with the best medical science throughout its facilities."

Additionally, Texas Christian's established a formal entity, the Evidence Based Outcomes Center (EBOC) that spearheads the organization's efforts to effectively use data to improve care and to make clinical practice consistent with the best medical science throughout its facilities. The EBOC develops evidence-based clinical guidelines designed to help Texas Children's clinicians manage the complexity of care and minimize variations in clinical practice — which results in improved quality. A multi-disciplinary team of experts at the EBOC develops the guidelines, which are then implemented into clinical practice.

The EBOC is tasked with:

> Identifying areas for quality improvement

> Assembling the right team to address guidelines for the targeted patient population

> Rigorously examining the latest clinical evidence

- Systematically creating guidelines with embedded recommendations and soliciting feedback from its community of clinical care users

- Teaming with clinical departments to roll out evidence-based guidelines to the broader clinician population

With the data aggregated in the TCH EDW for analytics purposes, the EBOC no longer has to cobble reports or manually analyze data. The EDW enables the EBOC to integrate data management, science through evidence, and then to effectively incorporate the evidence base into everyday clinical practice. These resources enable them to unlock the potential of their data, provide transparency to providers and mobilize clinicians to embrace quality improvement initiatives.

The team was able to efficiently identify areas with the most potential for quality improvement. Rather than needing six months to develop a clinical improvement initiative, EBOC could define patient cohorts, analyze baseline data, address data quality issues and define targeted improvement goals in 90 days. But this 50 percent improvement in process time was just the beginning. By subsequently implementing the Health Catalyst Population Explorer application, Texas Children's was able to far outdo even that distinct improvement, reducing the time to just two weeks.

Population Explorer, a foundational analytics application, is designed to accelerate development of clinical program improvements by delivering starter sets that consist of registries and a library of commonly defined measures. The EBOC team has leveraged 45 registries to date. Each of the registries, on average, includes 65 healthcare analytics measurements.

In addition to the registries and library of measures, these analytical tools provide the EBOC with:

- A platform upon which additional populations can be rapidly developed across the organization. The clinical improvement teams no longer have to start from scratch to define a target patient population. Instead, the team can identify and scope short-term and future projects quickly — a significant factor in reducing the time required to develop new clinical program improvement initiatives.

- Early identification of potential high-level data quality issues, such as missing data and inconsistent documentation. Data quality issues that are identified and addressed early help reduce the overall AIM Statement definition project phase timelines.

- More than 65 healthcare analytical measurements for each of the population registries. Each registry includes a common set of measurements — such as diagnosis, length of stay, case counts, demographics and readmission rates — that enable the clinical improvement teams to view metrics about individual patient populations. In addition to these common measurements, each registry features custom measurements based on labs, flow sheet data, vital signs, medications and other data appropriate to the registry.

⊙ Customizable drill-down data visualizations. Rather than having to sift through data and cobble together reports, EBOC teams receive actionable, timely insights through a variety of data visualizations. A sample Population Explorer visualization is shown in Figure 98.

Historically, identifying care improvement opportunities that would have the greatest impact was a challenge for Texas Children's. The Health Catalyst Key Process Analysis (KPA) application helped the hospital prioritize its quality improvement programs. Based on Pareto analysis — a statistical technique that identifies the limited number of tasks that will produce the most significant overall effect — the KPA application analyzed EDW data to pinpoint variability in care and areas of high resource consumption throughout the hospital.

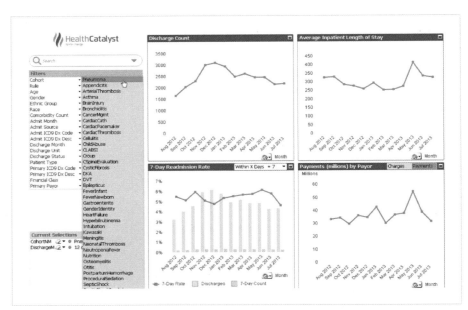

Figure 98: Sample Population Explorer visualization
(View Appendix C for larger version)

With this analysis in hand, Texas Children's decided to begin its quality improvement efforts by focusing on asthma care. Asthma is the most common chronic disease among children. In fact, an estimated 80,000 children in Houston alone suffer from asthma. In 2011, asthma accounted for 3,000 emergency department (ED) visits and 800 hospital admissions at Texas Children's.

As a first step toward better managing its asthma population, TCH established a cross-functional workgroup — called a clinical improvement team — consisting of physicians and nurses on the frontlines of care, as well as experts in patient safety, quality improvement, finance and information technology. This team was assigned to assess and manage acute asthma from the time of arrival in the ED to discharge.

Specifically, the team needed to determine how to pragmatically improve asthma care across hospital facilities. Texas Children's EBOC was on hand to support the team as it explored and implemented clinical best practices.

Using the wealth of new data at its disposal, the team built an asthma dashboard illustrated in Figure 99. Early in project, the improvement team discovered that a high volume of chest X-rays was being administered to asthma patients within the hospital. Rather than request an analyst's report to explain the cause, as they would have in the past, the team used the EDW's dashboards to immediately drill down into near real-time chest

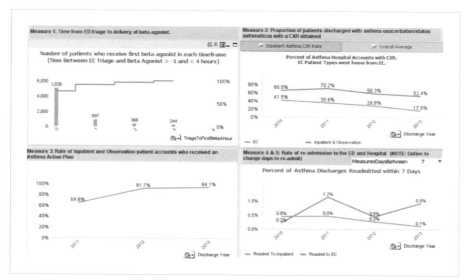

Figure 99: Sample asthma visualization
(View Appendix C for larger version)

X-ray data. To their astonishment, they recognized that, as a group, Texas Children's physicians were ordering chest X-rays for 65 percent of their asthma patients — when evidence-based practice calls for much lower usage of chest X-rays.

The workgroup traced the problem to a faulty order set within the hospital's EHR. Working with EBOC experts, the team developed a best practice for the order set, and the IT experts quickly rewrote the order set to reflect it.

Results

Pinpointing concrete opportunities for improvement is a significant achievement but actually driving adoption of better care-delivery practices is an often difficult prospect. Thanks to the cross-functional team approach that involves clinicians on the frontlines of care from the outset when determining the best ways to improve care delivery, Texas Children's was able to drive significant adoption and measurable results.

- ❯ Drove significant, measurable adoption of evidence-based order sets. Texas Children's focused on promoting appropriate chest X-ray orders for asthma patients among its hospitalist group. Today, Texas Children's physicians in the acute-care setting apply this evidence-based order set to approximately 80 percent of the asthma patients they treat. This represents a 67 percent increase — sustained for more than 8 months.

- ❯ Decreased inpatient length of stay (LOS) for asthma patients by 11 hours. By utilizing evidence-based practice across the continuum of care, Texas Children's was able to significantly decrease LOS for these patients as compared to the prior year.

- ⊗ Achieved and sustained a 49 percent decrease in unnecessary chest X-ray orders. Within six months, the number of chest X-rays ordered for asthma patients had declined by 15 percent. Today, these orders have decreased by 49 percent.

- ⊗ Sustained 67% increase in order set utilization. Today, 80% of all providers utilize evidence-based order sets, a 67% sustained increase over 8 months.

- ⊗ Increased use of an EHR-based asthma action plan by 90 percent of physicians. In conjunction with the EBOC, the clinical improvement team developed evidence-based asthma action plans for clinicians to provide to patients and families. These plans are designed to help patients better manage their asthma and recognize when clinical intervention is required. Today, 90 percent of physicians treating asthma patients are distributing these action plans.

- ⊗ Established an effective, permanent clinical improvement team that continues to identify areas for care improvement and build evidence-based practices into the care delivery workflow. Because the clinical improvement team owns improvement for one particular care family — asthma — over the long-term, they were able to standardize excellence in this care delivery work process. They have since turned their attention to optimizing additional work processes. For example, they are now working to reduce the delay between the time a child walks into the ED and the time they receive the appropriate asthma medications.

The discovery of the prevalent, unnecessary use of X-rays was an early win for Texas Children's to reduce unsafe testing and excess resource use and to align more fully with evidence-based care guidelines. This early success with asthma has encouraged Texas Children's to expand its improvement efforts to include multiple medical and surgical programs and processes, including appendectomy, diabetic ketoacidosis and more. The hospital even plans to expand the program beyond hospital-based care to include its primary pediatric practices and clinic-based care.

Reducing mortality from septicemia

Background

Leaders at MultiCare Health System (MultiCare), a Tacoma, Washington based health system, embarked on a journey to reduce mortality from septicemia. The effort was supported by the health system's top leadership who participated in a data driven approach to prioritize care improvement based on an analysis of resources consumed and variation in care outcomes.

Reducing septicemia mortality rates was identified as a top priority for MultiCare as a result of data that demonstrated three MultiCare hospitals were performing below national septicemia mortality averages and one additional hospital was performing well below those national averages.

In September, 2010, MultiCare implemented Health Catalyst's EDW and the three system approach for effective care delivery to measure and improve care through organizational and process improvements.

The EDW organized and simplified data from multiple data sources across the continuum of care. It became the single source of truth required to view care improvement opportunities and to measure change. It also proved to be an important means to unify clinical, information technology and financial leaders to collaboratively use clinical, operational and financial data to drive accountability for performance improvement.

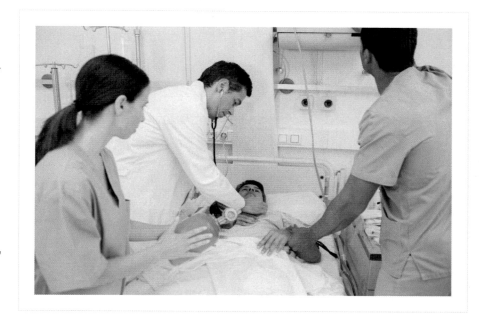

The first step in the process was to refine the clinical definition of sepsis. In the past, sepsis had proven difficult to define due to the complex comorbidity factors leading to septicemia. Using data from the EDW, leaders at MultiCare were able to explore around the boundaries of the definition and to ultimately settle on an algorithm that defined a septic patient. The iterative work resulted in increased confidence in the identified severe sepsis cohort.

The system-wide establishment and collaborative efforts of permanent, integrated teams consisting of clinicians, technologists, analysts and quality personnel was essential for accelerating MultiCare's efforts to reduce septicemia mortality. Together the collaborative addressed three key bodies of work — standard of care definition, early identification and efficient delivery of a defined care standard for septicemia.

The system-wide critical care collaborative streamlined several sepsis order sets from across the organization into one system-wide standard for the care of severely septic patients. Adult patients presenting with sepsis received the same care, no matter which MultiCare hospital they went to.

The critical care collaborative also worked to ensure timely implementation of the clinician defined standard of care to the sepsis cohort. The team used the code process that is commonly used in healthcare. Similar to other code processes (code trauma, code neuro, code STEMI, code sepsis) in use at MultiCare, the code sepsis designation was designed to bring together essential caregivers, in order to efficiently deliver time-sensitive, life-saving treatments to the patient presenting with severe sepsis.

> In just twelve months, MultiCare was able to reduce septicemia mortality rates by an average of 22 percent, leading to more than $1.3 million in validated cost savings during that same period.

Results

In just twelve months, MultiCare was able to reduce septicemia mortality rates by an average of 22 percent, leading to more than $1.3 million in validated cost savings during that same period. The sepsis cost reductions and quality of care improvements raised the expectation that similar results could be realized in other clinical conditions including heart failure, emergency department performance and inpatient throughput.

Reducing heart failure readmission rates

Background

Like most healthcare systems facing the transition to value-based reimbursement, a large, internationally renowned medical center found it necessary to assess its overall quality improvement program, with an emphasis on evaluating its data management capabilities.

Leadership realized it needed to be able to analyze and better manage specific patient populations, especially patients with chronic conditions and those at greatest risk for readmission. Administrators also recognized the need to address inefficiency and waste in the center's care programs, but they lacked hard data to confirm suspected problems or to detect hidden inefficiencies and safety issues.

To solve this problem, the medical center initially decided to deploy a traditional EDW based on the enterprise data model. However, it found that this type of EDW took years to fully deploy and failed to enable the near-real-time analysis of clinical data required for success under value-based care. The center then turned to Health Catalyst's Late-Binding™ Data Warehouse.

The new healthcare EDW was launched in mid-2011 and was fully deployed within just three months. The EDW quickly pooled financial, operational, patient satisfaction and clinical data from the center's EHR and other major applications. Then a multidisciplinary team of physicians, nurses and leaders from quality, finance, information technology and other medical center departments analyzed the pooled data using the Health Catalyst KPA application. The KPA application helped to pinpoint clinical areas with the highest variation that consume the most resources. It quickly identified cardiovascular as one of the top clinical programs with the greatest opportunity for improvement.

Armed with that insight and its new technology capabilities, the center applied for and received a grant from a major foundation to support a transitional care program for heart failure (HF) patients. The center borrowed the grant's objectives to define its long-term AIM Statement:

> AIM Statement:
> *To achieve and sustain a 30 percent reduction in the 30-day and a 15 percent reduction in the 90-day all-cause readmission rates for patients with heart failure by October 2014 and sustained reduction in readmission rates through 2016.*

> *To achieve and sustain a 30 percent reduction in the 30-day and a 15 percent reduction in the 90-day all-cause readmission rates for patients with heart failure by October 2014 and sustained reduction in readmission rates through 2016.*

Heart failure consistently ranks among the top five causes of hospital readmissions. According to the Centers for Medicare and Medicaid Services, Medicare Quality Hospital Chart Book (2011), during a recent three-year period the national rate of readmission for congestive heart failure was 24.7 percent, resulting in billions of dollars in direct medical costs.

To achieve the goals set forth in its AIM Statement, the center's clinical leaders developed three evidence-based, HF interventions, which were rolled out over a few months:

- Medication reconciliation – Within forty-eight hours of discharge, a physician reviews a list of the patient's medications with explicit instructions on how to properly take them.

- Post-discharge appointments – Before being discharged, patients are scheduled for follow-up care. When possible, patients at high risk for readmission are scheduled to be seen in the clinic within seven days of discharge. All others are scheduled to be seen within 14 days.

- Post-discharge phone calls – Within a specified time frame following discharge (again based on the patient's level of risk for readmission), a member from the coordinated care team calls patients to assess their condition and see if they have any questions or are having any problems with their medications.

As illustrated in Figure 100, an integrated dashboard was created in the healthcare analytical platform so clinicians and administrators could easily visualize the impact the process changes were having on readmissions. Additionally, the healthcare EDW and advanced HF analytics application allowed the multi-disciplinary teams to assess the interventions' impact on, costs and patient satisfaction.

To ensure that the focus on reducing readmissions did not have an unintentional effect in other areas, such as an increase in ED visits or a decrease in patient satisfaction, the center built in balance measures including the tracking of ED encounters, observation stays, length of stay and patient satisfaction rates.

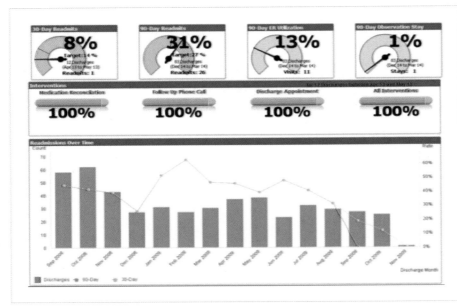

Figure 100: Sample heart failure readmission visualization
(View Appendix C for larger version)

Results

Six months after implementing the program, the medical center had experienced gratifying results including:

- A 63 percent increase in post-discharge physician medication reconciliation within 48 hours

- A two-fold increase in the number of phone calls made to patients within 48 hours of discharge

- A 21 percent seasonally adjusted reduction in 30-day HF readmissions

- A 14 percent seasonally adjusted reduction in 90-day HF readmissions

As a result of these successes, the medical center is extending the healthcare EDW deployment and quality intervention process within a community care program.

Improving Women and Newborns care

Background

Like many health systems, North Memorial Health Care in the Midwest metropolitan area of Minneapolis-St. Paul, Minnesota, has spent the last few years battling for financial stability. The 518-bed two-hospital system has struggled with rising costs, stiff regional pressures from an abundance of formidable competitors, and unpredictable reimbursement amid an uncertain political environment. To make matters worse, the health system was having difficulty collecting and analyzing data from its myriad information technology systems, leaving hospital leaders with an incomplete view of their financial pain points and opportunities for improvement.

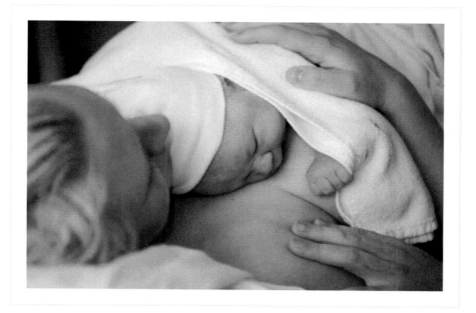

Amid these difficult market conditions, North Memorial's leadership determined to chart a path to sustainability. The many tactics they considered had one common thread — all relied on clinical and operational insight that could only come from aggregating data from the health system's EHR and other critical operational and financial information technology systems. A search for solutions to accomplish this task led to a decision to implement an adaptive, flexible, EDW platform with a data driven quality improvement program.

After using its newly implemented analytic system to analyze its total resources consumed, variation in care and cultural readiness, North Memorial's leadership selected the Women and Newborns department as the first target for quality improvement process. Within the department, the health system identified elective deliveries occurring prior to 39 weeks of gestation as the care process with the greatest opportunity for improvement and financial return. OB studies have shown that elective deliveries before 39 weeks increase the risk of newborn respiratory distress as well as increase the rates of C-sections where there is a higher rate of postpartum anemia and longer lengths-of-stay for both mothers and babies. Further incentive for focusing on early-term deliveries came from a savings agreement with a payer partner that promised to pay North Memorial a significant bonus in return for lowering its rate of pre-39-week deliveries by half, from 1.2 percent of all deliveries to 0.6 percent.

This project was also one that North Memorial could set up and launch very quickly. Reducing deliveries before 39 weeks was an excellent launch point because there is significant peer-reviewed research in this area. If they solved this problem, the scale of the services would allow clinicians to significantly improve care as well as reduce costs quickly.

To begin their work on early-term deliveries, North Memorial established a service line guidance team comprised of OB/GYN specialists, primary care physicians, nurses, data architects and outcomes analysts, all led by Dr. Jon Nielsen, the director of Women and Newborns services at North Memorial. Their job was to define when pre-term deliveries were appropriate, standardize workflow and create improved processes for pregnant women and newborn care.

The new team's first effort was to load a subset of North Memorial's data to analyze existing workflow issues and performance measures. Once they had a clear picture of the problem in hand, the team decided to implement a new process for managing elective pre-39-week deliveries. Previously, elective deliveries were relatively easy for nurses to approve and schedule. The new process embedded in the EHR workflow still allowed nurses to schedule pre-term deliveries, but only if they passed a checklist of requirements for medical necessity. Elective deliveries were immediately referred to the Women and Newborns chair for review.

> The percentage of all deliveries that were elective pre-39-week surgeries plummeted from 1.2 percent to just 0.3 percent, shattering the payer's goal of 0.6 percent and earning North Memorial a six-figure bonus payment.

As with any quality improvement initiative, North Memorial had to overcome physician resistance to the changes in Women and Newborns care. True data-driven decision-making was something new for many clinicians.

To win physicians over, clinical leaders attended multiple staff meetings to explain the reasoning behind the process changes for pre-term deliveries, and to share the supporting data. Gradually, North Memorial's physicians began to see the importance of following the new guidelines. North Memorial accelerated the transformation by appealing to physicians' competitive natures. Each North Memorial clinic posted internal provider report cards indicating the number of elective pre-39-week deliveries approved by each provider. Physicians began to change their practice patterns when they saw their performance being compared to peers.

Results

North Memorial's use of data from its newly implemented analytic, deployment and content systems reduced the health system's rate of elective pre-term deliveries by 75 percent in just six months. The percentage of all deliveries that were elective pre-39-week surgeries plummeted from 1.2 percent to just 0.3 percent, shattering the payer's goal of 0.6 percent and earning North Memorial a six-figure bonus payment.

The results of this project were so promising that North Memorial has since approached other insurers in the Twin Cities about entering into shared cost-reduction reimbursement contracts for additional care processes. This early improvement project proved their ability to reduce complications and NICU admissions for newborns, saving money for insurers and employers. Going forward, North Memorial leaders are optimistic that both groups will agree to reward them for delivering ever higher quality at reduced costs, as it aligns perfectly with the emerging national focus on value-based purchasing.

Improving hospital acquired infection surveillance

Background

All healthcare systems face the same dual challenge. They need to wring out expenses at the same time that government is imposing new regulatory challenges — not the least of which are increased Hospital Acquired Infection (HAI) reporting requirements.

A large medical center needed to streamline its process for identifying patients with central-line associated bloodstream infections (CLABSI) and catheter-associated urinary tract infections (CAUTI). These nosocomial (e.g., hospital-acquired) infections are associated with longer patient stays, increased mortality, as well as increased care costs — an estimated $20,000 per CLABSI case. Furthermore, they are largely preventable.

Clinical resources that might have been directed to improving patient care were spent manually tracking lab results and reviewing data to determine if patients' positive blood or urine cultures correlated to nosocomial infections.

In order to mine and display their data, the health system utilized an advanced application on top of their EDW that included automated clinical algorithms that adhere to National Healthcare Safety Network (NHSN) definitions. The algorithms provide inclusion and exclusion criteria for patients. For algorithm validation, all cultures processed by the hospital, were collected in a retrospective electronic search for a six-month time period. These results were validated utilizing NHSN surveillance definitions by trained infection preventionists in a thorough chart review.

Results

Within six months, chart reviews showed that use of the HAI surveillance application delivered more accurate regulatory reporting of HAI rates with a 90% reduction in surveillance resources. In addition, it supported a near real-time reporting dashboard that displayed analytics in a highly visual, easy-to-interpret display, as illustrated in Figure 101.

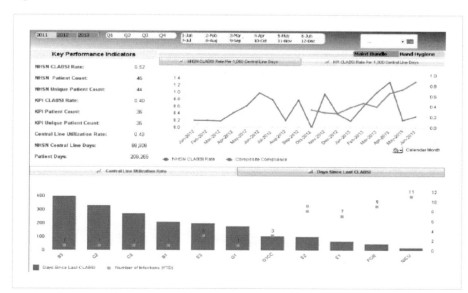

Figure 101: Sample CLABSI visualization
(View Appendix C for larger version)

The net effect is that infection preventionists now spend far more time focusing on education, clinical interventions and analysis versus time consuming chart reviews by hand. Over time these interventions have contributed to decreasing infection rates.

A multi-disciplinary team including infection preventionists, clinicians, technical, financial, quality and clinical improvement departments worked together to evaluate the hospital's quality measures, identify HAI opportunities for improvement, revise the EDW's algorithms, and to develop easy-to-understand visualizations. Past initiatives of this type tended to be of a temporary nature. Today this team meets on a monthly basis to ensure the clinical improvement gains are sustained and to evaluate opportunities for expansion into additional care process families such as septicemia.

The EDW's impact is being felt well beyond HAI surveillance and improved detection rates. The medical center has developed five steams of quality improvement — infectious disease, population health, cardiovascular, neuroscience and oncology.

Streamlining operations

Before implementing the EDW, Pediatric Radiology and other departments throughout the health system relied on an inefficient, time-consuming process to generate operational reports for internal reporting purposes. In fact, practice administrators and even senior leadership like assistant directors throughout Texas Children's had to dedicate several hours a week to manual analysis for weekly or biweekly reporting — interfering significantly with time spent on other operational responsibilities and analysis of the data.

For Pediatric Radiology, creating such reports involved requesting data from the radiology Information Systems (IS) manager. Significant discussion between operations and IS personnel was required to determine which data was needed. The IS manager would have to manually extract the needed data from the EHR database. She would then send the data to the radiology practice administrator in an Excel spreadsheet containing as many as 300,000 rows of data.

At this point, the radiology practice administrator had to spend valuable time researching and making sense of the data, slicing and dicing it to build reports and analyzing different variables. The difficulty of this task was compounded by the fact that a lot of important data was simply missing. For example, Pediatric Radiology lacked information on referrals, utilization metrics and diagnosis codes related to imaging procedures. In addition, the administrator had to work with the data further to create charts and graphs in a PowerPoint format for executive presentations.

Radiology was only one of many departments throughout the health system that would have to repeat this time-consuming process on a regular basis. To streamline the process and enable better operational insights, Texas Children's decided to implement Health Catalyst's Operational Advanced Application–Radiology Module to run on its EDW platform. The health system had already deployed several advanced analytics applications on the EDW platform to drive clinical quality improvement. They were confident they could drive similar improvements on an operational front.

Results

Pediatric Radiology now has baseline data they can share quickly with senior management in a graphical, easy-to-understand format, as shown in Figure 102. The data includes process metrics such as:

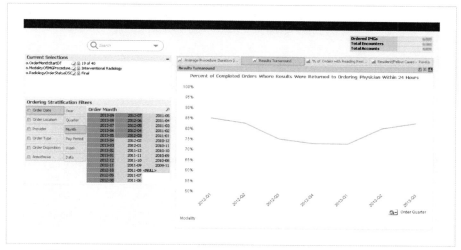

Figure 102: Sample provider results turnaround visualization
(View Appendix C for larger version)

- ❯ Average procedure duration

- ❯ Results turnaround time to providers

- ❯ Percentage of orders with reading residents

- ❯ Anesthesia utilization

- ❯ Resident or fellow cases

- ❯ Patient flow cycle time (including check-in to exam, check-in to results, end of exam to results, exam begin to exam end, and percent of appointments cancelled)

Having this data and established baselines enables the department to target process improvement efforts that help drive improved patient and provider satisfaction.

The ability to generate reports easily and immediately has saved the organization an estimated $400,000 and has freed up operations personnel to focus on important strategic and operational matters. The new process eliminates frustrations between IS and operations personnel because IS no longer has to perform regular manual reporting. The EDW solution enables the practice administrator to self-serve — accessing near-real-time data to make highly informed operational decisions. This automated, efficient process eliminates the "fire drill mentality" that consumes so many resources.

The EDW platform has also delivered insights to Pediatric Radiology that are helping the group improve care delivery, prevent service leakage and increase provider and patient satisfaction. Examples of results and opportunities for improved delivery of care and patient satisfaction include:

- Pediatric Radiology can now track process metrics such as the time it takes to get results to a provider after an order is completed. The analytics application alerted the team to a decline in their performance on this metric. This information enabled them to address the delay issues, and they are now tracking back up at 85 percent for provider results turnaround time. The ability for providers to obtain this clinical information quickly helps facilitate timely care delivery.

- Pediatric Radiology can now track the time between patient check-in and exam start time. TCH has established a baseline for this metric that will help them understand their patient satisfaction as it relates to wait time.

The EDW data has also helped Pediatric Radiology drive cost improvement. As described previously, moving from a manual process to automated, near-real-time reporting has driven significant efficiencies and dollar savings. The practice has also been able to reduce and avoid waste. For example, they are tracking anesthesia utilization to ensure appropriate, cost-effective use. They are also tracking their utilization of each piece of equipment — a process that has shown them where they have additional capacity so they can move volume around the system to maximize utilization and reduce scheduling lags.

EDW analysis has enabled the group to increase revenue by minimizing procedure referral leakage. The health system recently acquired two obstetrics physician groups that weren't referring to Texas Children's Pediatric Radiology. The advanced analytics application allowed the department to analyze both groups' orders — what they were ordering from Texas Children's and what they weren't — by modality and clinical indication. From this, they were able to extract the imaging procedures they didn't provide and easily determine which referrals they should have been receiving. After the department presented this data to the two groups, new referrals began flowing in immediately. Texas Children's estimates they have gained $1 million in billable charges as a result of this effort and they have improved the delivery of patient care with an integrated patient healthcare record.

> "Texas Children's estimates they have gained $1 million in billable charges as a result of this effort and they have improved the delivery of patient care with an integrated patient healthcare record."

Finally, the availability of data in the EDW has streamlined internal processes like budgeting. In the past, the yearly budgeting process required spending several days getting operations and finance personnel on the same page. It might take days of discussion just to agree on the definition of a radiology unit of measure for volume. Now all teams use the same vernacular and measurements, making the process more efficient and focused on strategic planning rather than definitions.

In conclusion

The examples presented in this chapter come from a variety of different organizations. Collectively, they provide a glimpse into the future: a future characterized by clinical and operational leaders using the three systems (analytic, deployment and content) to continuously improve processes in pursuit of clinical and operational excellence. In the not-so-distant future, these types of improvement initiatives will be the norm. Clinicians will truly be managing the process of care. We are entering into a new era in healthcare. Organizations who embrace the three system framework will be positioned for a new future characterized by new models of care delivery and population health management, which are discussed in the next chapter.

> " We are entering into a new era in healthcare. Organizations who embrace the three system framework will be positioned for a new future characterized by new models of care delivery and population health management ... "

8 INNOVATION IN HEALTHCARE: CREATING TOMORROW

In this chapter we share trends and technologies that promise to transform healthcare and discuss the implication of these trends for healthcare analytics.

"I haven't failed. I have just found 10,000 ways that won't work."
– *Thomas Edison*

"Don't be afraid to fail. Be afraid not to try." – Michael Jordan

While this book has many objectives, the primary goal is to stimulate a new way of thinking about healthcare. Over the past century, we have made tremendous progress in our ability to help patients. However, many challenges still remain. Healthcare transformation is a demanding endeavor. The good news is that it is possible to get a sense of what the new world will look like and start creating a new vision for the future of care.

> Patient care has made astonishing advances over the past several decades. However, there is also no doubt that healthcare in the U.S. — and in most other countries — is ailing and in need of help.

Patient care has made astonishing advances over the past several decades. However, there is also no doubt that healthcare in the U.S. — and in most other countries — is ailing and in need of help. Too often, the packaging and delivery of treatment are inefficient, ineffective and not patient friendly. Problems range from medical errors — which according to the Institute of Medicine (IOM) represent the eighth-leading cause of death in the U.S. — to poor outcomes and soaring costs. Astonishingly, one-fourth of the U.S. gross domestic product is spent on healthcare. Healthcare inflation continues to grow much faster than the economy, and it threatens the economic future of our governments, businesses and individual citizens. We must focus more on other determinants of health — beyond clinical care delivery — if we are to make progress in improving the health of populations, enhancing patient satisfaction and reducing costs. These issues require innovative and highly collaborative solutions involving all stakeholders (e.g., clinicians, community, patients, operational leaders, payers, IT and policymakers). These new solutions need to encompass every aspect of healthcare, from delivery to patients, to its technology, and its business and care models. Now is the time for creativity.

The role of innovation

Our world faces major healthcare, economic, environmental and social challenges. While no single approach holds all the answers, innovation is a key element in any effort to improve people's lives. As organizations and countries strive to improve productivity, enhance quality and ensure sustained growth, they will need to boost their capacity to innovate. Innovation is essential for addressing some of society's most pressing issues, such as climate change, poverty and health.

Innovation can be defined in many ways. Innovation represents something new, original or improved that creates value for people. It generally refers to renewing, changing or creating more effective processes, products or services. For organizations, this means implementing new ideas, creating dynamic products or improving existing services. Innovation can be a catalyst for organizational growth and success by helping the organization to adapt in a competitive marketplace.

Being innovative does not necessarily mean inventing something. Innovation can mean changing an organization's business model and adapting to changes in an organization's environment to deliver better products or services. Successful innovation should be an integral part of an organization's business strategy as it endeavors to be a leader in original thinking and creative problem solving.

In healthcare, the term, innovation, has traditionally been reserved for the development of new diagnostic procedures, therapies, drugs or medical devices — something the U.S. has excelled in over the past few decades. From checklists to surgical robots, new approaches to healthcare continue to make their way into practice — with some stunning results.

> " Being innovative does not necessarily mean inventing something. Innovation can mean changing an organization's business model and adapting to changes in an organization's environment to deliver better products or services. "

There is a litany of emerging technologies that promise to have a profound impact on healthcare in the future, including minimally invasive surgery, drug delivery systems, monitoring sensors, organ assistance devices, stem cell technologies, genomics, imaging technologies, 3D printing, tissue and fluid bioengineering, nanotechnology, mobile computing technologies, robotics, regenerative medicine, remote patient management systems, telehealth, wireless technologies and information technology systems, to name a few. The list of healthcare innovation possibilities is long and steadily growing.

As both private and public efforts to reform the U.S. healthcare system gain momentum, it is clear that innovation must encompass more than just new medical devices or products. Innovation needs to explore new areas, including delivery system organization, care model design, data analytics, patient engagement and provider incentives.

Population Health — moving beyond random acts to a comprehensive approach

A significant portion of this book has focused on building the necessary systems and capabilities to create scalable and sustainable data-driven change to ensure future success. Organizations, like human beings, need to learn to walk before they run. The end point, however, mandates that organizations move beyond what nationally known physician executive and quality advocate Jim Reinertsen, MD, calls "random acts of improvement" to comprehensively managing the health and well-being of patient populations. This is not to suggest that improving individual patient care processes is unimportant or unnecessary. It definitely is. However, healthcare organizations need to improve both individual patient care processes and, at the same time, learn to manage the health of the entire population of patients they serve.

David Kindig and Greg Stoddard define population health as "the health outcomes of a group of individuals, including the distribution of such outcomes within the group."[105] The goal of population health is to improve the health and well-being of an entire population of people. Clinical care certainly plays a role in population health, but success also requires reducing health inequities and disparities among population groups and addressing the social, environmental and genetic determinants of health that we discussed in chapter 1.

> Successfully addressing population health requires focusing on the broader population instead of focusing solely on individual patient care processes. It requires a "both–and," not an "either–or" approach.

Successfully addressing population health requires focusing on the broader population instead of focusing solely on individual patient care processes. It requires a "both–and," not an "either–or" approach. Population health addresses a comprehensive set of factors that have been demonstrated to impact the health of individuals and populations. The World Health Organization (WHO) indicates that these social determinants of health are responsible for the bulk of diseases and injuries and are the major cause of health inequities in all countries of the world.[106] In the United States, social determinants of health are estimated to account for 70 percent of avoidable mortality.[107]

From a population health perspective, health has been defined not simply as a state free from disease and injury, but as "the capacity of people to adapt to, respond to or control life's challenges and changes."[108] The WHO has defined health broadly as "a state of complete physical, mental, and social well-being and not merely the absence of disease or infirmity."[109, 110] Healthcare providers need to focus on this broader perspective as we shift our focus to value and maintaining the health and well-being of populations of patients.

Engaging healthcare providers in population health improvement is critical because functional status and quality of life are ultimately what matter most to patients. While present-day clinical care contributes to health, health outcomes are directly impacted by the prevalence of unhealthy behaviors — in addition to the incidence of disease. Furthermore, the steadily rising incidence of chronic diseases, exacerbated by unhealthy behaviors, is the single biggest contributor to the growth of healthcare costs. An effective strategy to improve health and assure long-term sustainable healthcare cost reductions requires healthcare providers to help individuals be as healthy as possible in their homes and communities.

Due to the fragmented healthcare market and disconnected information systems, no single provider group can improve population health on its own. Integration of skills and services is required, along with effective leadership, to assure that various stakeholders come together in a collaborative fashion. Healthcare providers play a prominent role in this endeavor, but they also have to collaborate with insurers, public health and community stakeholders.

In an era of accelerating change, healthcare providers have understandably focused on improving individual patient care processes and lowering costs. This is a natural and expected approach. However, increasing the value of healthcare on a broader scale — that is, improving population health while reducing the high costs of the care delivery system — is far more challenging. Large regional care delivery systems provide care to individual patients and populations over many years. The longer the time span, the greater the number of healthcare settings and clinicians who are involved in a patient's care. Achieving significantly better outcomes requires collaboration between providers and stakeholders in a community as well as the three systems (analytic, deployment and content) discussed in chapter 3. Data-driven population management is a natural extension of an organization's improvement activities, albeit an order of magnitude more complex.

Still, effective population management is a worthy goal. Longitudinal improvements in care delivery and efficiency offer the greatest potential for reducing morbidity, eliminating inappropriate variation, reducing health disparities, eradicating waste and improving quality of life.

The emerging era of healthcare demands a more effective focus on population health. There is no better time for innovation in population health than now.

Critical innovations that promise to transform medicine

As we have discussed, healthcare innovations range from the process of care to models of care, to how healthcare organizations are organized, to key technological advances that support population health. Let's turn our attention to a few key areas of innovation that promise to transform healthcare over the next few years — and those that will have significant implications for the future of healthcare analytics.

> Due to the fragmented healthcare market and disconnected information systems, no single provider group can improve population health on its own. Integration of skills and services is required, along with effective leadership, to assure that various stakeholders come together in a collaborative fashion.

Value is becoming healthcare's new mantra. We are shifting from simply doing things to a system based on outcomes and value production that encompasses the individual patient, populations and communities. At first glance, achieving value in healthcare might seem straightforward and easy. And yet it is actually complex and difficult, particularly when attempted on a broad scale, such as the health of an entire population over many years.

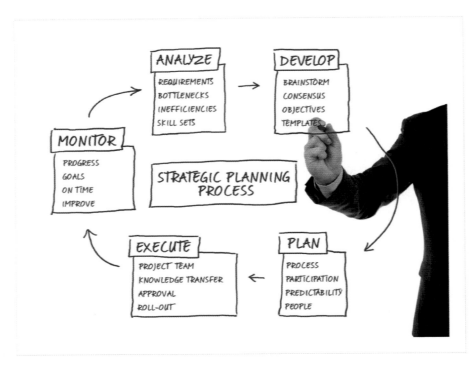

Achieving value in healthcare and successfully managing the health of populations requires a wide range of interested parties to center on the things they hold most dear — most notably the health and well-being of the patients they serve. Future success mandates achieving a collection of important goals that collectively lead to improved outcomes and reduced costs: coordination of care, improved efficiencies, patient centeredness and effective population management. Every healthcare organization's future success depends on achieving these high-value goals. Thomas Lee, MD, talking about healthcare value, said that "no one can oppose this goal and expect long-term success."[111]

It is unclear whether the value movement can foster the fundamental changes required to transform the healthcare industry. While achieving value has appeal, it also requires overcoming some daunting clinical, operational and organizational challenges. Value suggests that providers learn how to treat patients as whole persons and develop outcome measures that stretch beyond encounter-specific indicators to account for all of a patient's or population's needs over time (i.e., for complete episodes of care), thereby producing more comprehensive measures that reflect the well-being of both patients and populations.

As the concept of healthcare value becomes more prominent, healthcare providers will have a beacon to move toward. The emphasis on the whole patient and on populations will encourage and require teamwork among clinicians and across specialties, as well as coordination among clinical care units and healthcare organizations of all types across the continuum of care (e.g., physician groups, hospitals, health systems, payers and vendors). This will require all parties to relinquish their traditional siloed views and adopt a more expansive and collaborative model of care delivery — one that respects the talent and experience brought to the table by all stakeholders. The need for this level of collaboration and coordination has led to the concept of the Accountable Care Organization (ACO).

The term Accountable Care Organization was first coined in 2006 by Elliott Fisher, M.D., Director of the Center for Health Policy Research at the Geisel School of Medicine at Dartmouth. The ACO concept immediately sparked a great deal of interest and debate. The interest gained additional momentum in 2009 when the Affordable Care Act (ACA) used a specific Centers for Medicare and Medicaid Services (CMS) drafted definition of an ACO. The following discussion focuses on the general ACO concept as defined by Fisher and others, versus the specific ACA definition.

While the ACO concept is still evolving, it is generically defined as a group of health care providers — potentially including doctors, hospitals, health plans and other health care constituents — who voluntarily come together to provide coordinated, high-quality care to populations of patients. The goal of the coordinated care provided by an ACO is to ensure that patients and populations — especially the chronically ill — get the right care at the right time and without harm, while avoiding care that has no proven benefit or represents an unnecessary duplication of services.

> The goal of the coordinated care provided by an ACO is to ensure that patients and populations — especially the chronically ill — get the right care at the right time and without harm, while avoiding care that has no proven benefit or represents an unnecessary duplication of services.

An ACO may use a range of payment models (e.g., fee for service, with or without shared savings arrangements; capitation for specific defined populations, such as diabetes; or global capitation, based on a payment per person, rather than a payment per service provided). The traditional transaction-based payment model does not provide the incentives required to support ACOs and population health. As the reimbursement model migrates toward payment for value, this will change. It is anticipated that ACOs will increasingly be reimbursed under a capitated model that incentivizes optimal quality, safety, efficiency and health outcomes for populations of patients.

ACOs are accountable to the patients they serve and to third-party payers for the quality, appropriateness, efficiency and safety of the healthcare they provide. In addition to attending to the ill and injured, providers who work under these plans need to focus on preventive healthcare since there is greater financial reward in preventing illness than in treatment. These plans dissuade providers from using expensive, newly developed treatment options that may be less effective or have only a marginally higher success rate versus time-honored alternatives.

Under capitation, healthcare providers assume part or all of traditional insurance risk. Revenues are fixed, and each patient enrolled in a capitated plan makes claims against the provider's total resources. By accepting a fixed payment, participating physicians essentially become the enrolled patients' insurers by resolving patients' claims at the point of care delivery. In doing so, physicians assume the responsibility for the patients' unknown future healthcare costs.

Large providers serve a larger population than do smaller providers. The increased population size of large providers allows them to more effectively manage variations in service requirements and costs — and hence manage risk better. However, even large ACOs may not be able to manage global risk as effectively as a large insurer. The populations managed by large insurers typically dwarf the population of existing provider-sponsored ACOs. As a result, the insurers' annual costs as a percentage of annual cash flow fluctuate far less than those of an ACO managing a much smaller population. In the case of ACOs with smaller patient populations, the potential variation in annual costs is greater, and the risk that costs could exceed a provider's annual revenues is larger. The smaller the population under a capitated agreement, the more likely that a relatively small number of costly patients can significantly affect a provider's costs and increase the provider's risk of insolvency.

> " An ACO consisting of physician groups and hospitals generally lacks the requisite accounting, actuarial, underwriting and financial experience and capability for managing risk. However, their most significant issue is the greater degree of variation in estimates of annual average patient costs. "

An ACO consisting of physician groups and hospitals generally lacks the requisite accounting, actuarial, underwriting and financial experience and capability for managing risk. However, their most significant issue is the greater degree of variation in estimates of annual average patient costs. This leaves the ACO at a significant financial disadvantage in comparison to insurers whose estimates of a population's risks and costs are far more accurate because of their larger sample size.[112] Because their risks are inversely related to the size of the population under their care, ACOs will inevitably try to increase the number of patients under their care in a capitated plan. This will incentivize mergers, acquisitions and growth. The only way an ACO can manage populations as effectively as a larger insurer is to achieve populations the size of a typical large insurer and incorporate the level of expertise and risk assessment characteristic of a large insurer.

ACOs could potentially be sponsored by a variety of existing types of healthcare provider organizations, including large physician groups, physician and hospital alliances (i.e., physician-hospital organizations, or PHOs), integrated delivery networks (IDNs) and independent practice associations (IPAs). All of these organizational entities possess management and organizational elements that are necessary to form an ACO. However, each typically falls short of the full expertise and infrastructure needed to assume the risk of managing populations and to achieve the cost structures required to succeed as an ACO.

Companies that implement accountable care need to be able to provide two important capabilities: population health management and accountable care administration, financing and risk management. Population health management includes the following:

❶ Creation of a care delivery network that can service a population of patients in a defensible area by assembling appropriate provider resources (e.g., primary care physicians, specialists, hospitals, etc.).

❷ Clinically defined populations of patients for which the organization is willing and able to assume risk.

> Companies that implement accountable care need to be able to provide two important capabilities: population health management and accountable care administration, financing and risk management.

❸ Systematic improvement in the quality of care being delivered to the defined populations and ensuring the appropriate amount of care is delivered.

❹ Systematic elimination of waste within the care delivery process: reductions in the cost per member per month.

Population health management excellence can be compared to acquiring and cutting a diamond. This capability becomes the ACO's most valuable asset — as represented by the diamond in Figure 103. In addition, the ACO also needs to package and effectively market its capabilities to payers of various types, using a combination of analytic, financial, marketing, risk assessment and negotiation tools and methods. This

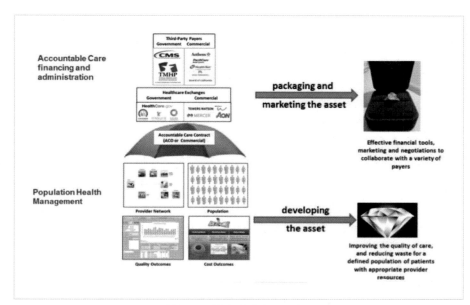

Figure 103: ACO model
(Click for larger version)

can be compared to placing the diamond in a gold setting and placing the completed ring in velvet-lined box, as shown in Figure 103. An effective ACO needs the diamond and the packaging.

An effective ACO needs to become a true system of care delivery capable of achieving high-quality medical outcomes in an efficient manner. This necessitates a level of alignment and integration among various constituents that has not historically been characteristic of healthcare. Realizing this goal requires overcoming a variety of significant barriers and challenges:

- ❯ Cultural. An effective ACO needs to be patient-centric and highly focused on the process of care. This requires that ACOs be clinician-led, or at least have a very strong patient and clinician voice. They also need to be self-reflective, focused on continuous improvement and flexible enough to manage a complex, adaptive system like a large ACO. Accomplishing full integration of the different cultures, services and constituents that comprise an ACO is not an easy task.

- ❯ Organizational structure. A successful ACO must have an effective organization capable of managing governance, provider recruitment and relations, enrollment, member services, population health, legal issues, costs and reimbursement.

- ❯ Clinical staff. An adequate number of primary care providers (PCPs) is essential. Given the national shortage of PCPs, this is difficult to achieve. Disparate medical specialties need to be aligned into a single medical group that, in close collaboration with its primary care peers, manages large populations of patients across the care continuum over many years. The large income disparities between specialties pose a challenge here. Finally, a highly collaborative, multidisciplinary team approach to care delivery is needed.

- ❯ Administrative resources. An effective ACO needs to have adequate staff, time and money to assume the responsibility of managing large populations of patients. A high degree of alignment and effective, efficient service delivery models need to be developed. ACOs need actuarial, underwriting and financial expertise to manage risk.

- ❯ Legal. Some ACOs may initially try to form and operate on a contractual basis. However, without migrating to a complete, fully integrated legal business entity, it will be difficult for these organizations to overcome the anti-trust, anti-kickback and self-referral laws and regulations that currently exist.

- ❯ Size. Successful ACOs have to achieve the critical mass, expertise and operating efficiency needed to manage the outcomes and risks of the large populations required for financial viability.

- **Prioritization.** In order to effectively focus scarce resources, ACOs need to be able to prioritize needs based on identifying high-risk patients and high-volume areas of inappropriate variation that significantly drive costs. Prioritization will help ACOs understand the areas that significantly impact costs and develop an effective payment structure strategy.

- **Market expertise.** Because healthcare markets can vary considerably, an effective ACO needs to fully understand its market position and competition. It must also be able to target customers, evaluate risk, establish appropriate provider networks and manage network access agreements.

- **Referral management.** An ACO needs a structure and process to effectively manage referrals to specialists, academic centers and other high-cost specialized care units.

- **Utilization management.** An ACO needs to effectively manage utilization, including patients with the highest utilization and costs, which usually means patients with chronic conditions.

- **Source data acquisition.** An ACO must acquire and integrate data from all participating constituents, including hospitals, employed physicians, affiliated physicians (not employed by the ACO), post-acute care (e.g., SNF, IRF/LTCH, home health, hospice) and payers. Hospital data comes from electronic health records (EHRs), financial, operational and patient satisfaction source systems, to name a few. Examples of payer data include claims, utilization and costs.

- **Quality metrics and analytics.** ACOs need to develop meaningful metrics for individual patient conditions (especially for chronic diseases) and for population health and well-being. This requires a highly sophisticated and flexible analytic system.

In order to be successful, an ACO must address these challenges. Most of these barriers and challenges will require the three systems for effective care delivery outlined in part 2 of this book: analytic, deployment and content.

Innovative, highly integrated delivery systems based on the ACO concept offer a great deal of promise, but achieving the vision of improved patient satisfaction, improved population health and reduced costs will take time, thought and hard work. A number of good references on ACOs (their purpose, future and challenges) can be found in the reference section.[113, 114]

> " Innovative, highly integrated delivery systems based on the ACO concept offer a great deal of promise, but achieving the vision of improved patient satisfaction, improved population health and reduced costs will take time, thought and hard work. "

Innovation in models of care — the medical home

The National Committee for Quality Assurance (NCQA) supported patient-centered medical home (PCMH) represents both a philosophy and a model of care delivery that is accessible, patient-centered, coordinated, holistic, multidisciplinary, team based and focused on quality, safety and prevention. In recent years, the concept has evolved into a widely accepted model for how primary care should be organized and delivered in health systems across the U.S.

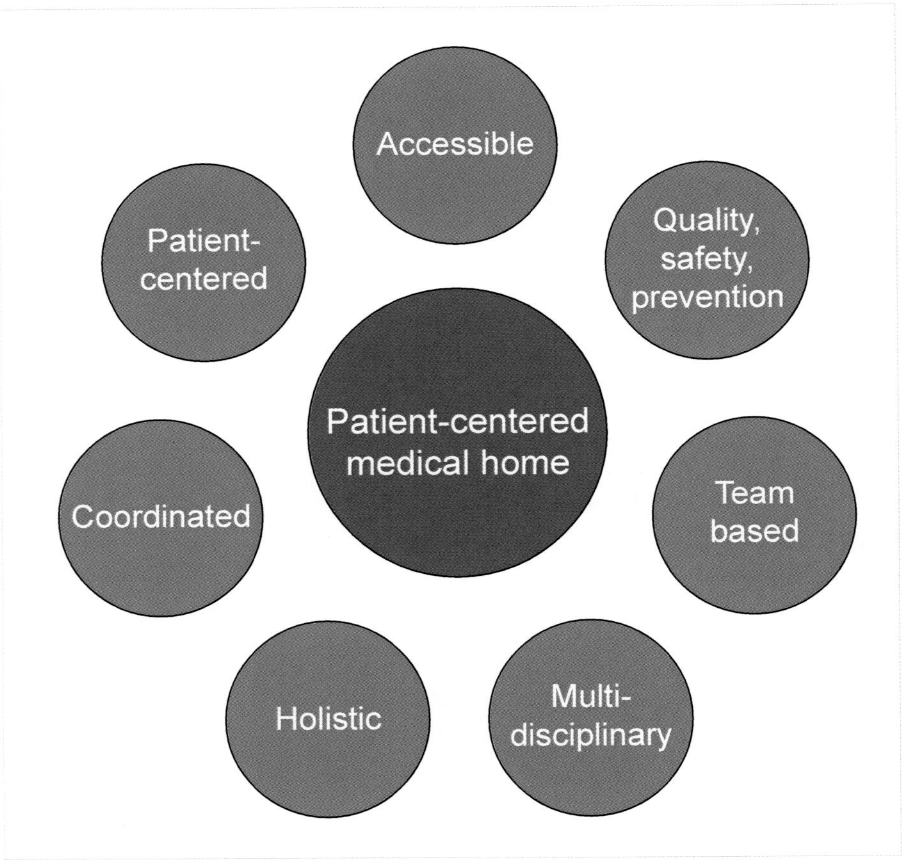

Figure 104: Patient-centered medical home

In 2007, the key primary care associations developed and adopted the Joint Principles of the Patient-Centered Medical Home to describe the characteristics of the PCMH.[115] The PCMH philosophy encourages providers and care teams to address the patients' healthcare needs — from simple to complex conditions — where they are (i.e., in their homes). It also promotes an environment of compassion, dignity and respect in an effort to build strong and trusting relationships between patients and providers. The PCMH does not represent a specific end point. Rather, it is a model for achieving care excellence with care delivered in the right place, at the right time and in a manner that is optimized for patients. A considerable amount of published evidence exists suggesting that the PCMH can be effective in improving patient outcomes.[116, 117, 118, 119, 120]

Along with ACOs, the PCMH plays an important role in the future coordination of patient care. The IOM suggests that the core functions of primary care consist of "accessible, comprehensive, longitudinal, and coordinated care in the context of families and community."[121]

The PCMH model encourages the full integration of all the services patients and families need. The patient is intimately involved in managing their care and in interpreting information regarding their care — while working in close collaboration with their care provider to develop a care plan that aligns with his or her needs, values and preferences.

Appropriate care for a patient or a population of patients depends on the characteristics and complexity of their needs. The challenges involved in delivering and managing their care increases as the complexity of their needs increases. These challenges include acute illness or injury, chronic illness, health-limiting behaviors, prevention requirements and the environment in which the patient lives. Additional factors include the patient's preferences and their ability to organize and participate in their care. A multidisciplinary care team is required to carefully coordinate and manage this level of complexity, whether it is an individual patient or a population of patients.

> "Appropriate care for a patient or a population of patients depends on the characteristics and complexity of their needs. The challenges involved in delivering and managing their care increases as the complexity of their needs increases."

ACOs that effectively use the PCMH model are better able to achieve two important objectives: high-quality and high-value care. ACOs that leverage the coordinated care provided by the PCMH model and facilitate good communication and a high level of coordinated care for their populations are better able to manage transitions of care and align the necessary resources to meet the care needs of the patients they serve. ACOs can also implement support systems that enable coordinated care in both ambulatory and non-ambulatory settings. With these support systems in place, care delivery is far more seamless than it is in our present, disjointed model of care delivery.

The PCMH is even more powerful when it is combined with the capabilities of health information technology (HIT) to enable rapid quality improvement. In order to realize this potential, ACOs need to implement the analytic, deployment and content systems described in chapters 3-6. HIT facilitates the PCMH in a variety of important ways:

- Collection, storage, management and exchange of relevant patient health information, including data generated and collected by the patient.

- Facilitation of communication between providers, care teams, patients and families to support more efficient and effective care delivery and care coordination.

- Collection, storage, measurement and analytics of individual patient and populations of patient outcomes in order to document and maximize the quality of care and other important outcomes.

- Real-time and retrospective decision support for clinicians.

- Patient engagement and facilitation of more effective self-management under the supervision of care teams.

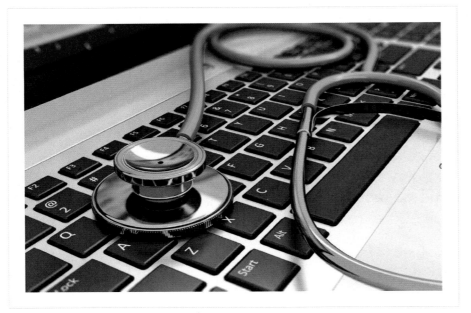

Clearly, HIT alone does not automatically create a fully functional PCMH. However, it can greatly augment one. At a minimum, a functional EHR, an enterprise data warehouse and healthcare analytics are required to support a PCMH. In addition, there are other technologies that can enhance and support an effective PCMH, including patient portals, remote patient management and telehealth technologies, and social networking media. Next, we will look at these technologies and their implications for healthcare analytics.

Transformational technologies and healthcare analytics

A number of emerging technologies promise to transform how, when and where care is delivered — and to significantly enhance diagnostic and therapeutic options for clinicians and patients. Let's consider some of these advances and their potential impact on analytics.

Creating value with patient portals

A patient portal is a secure website that provides patients 24-hour access to their personal health information from anywhere. A well-designed patient portal provides patients with the opportunity to interact with their healthcare provider and to participate in their health decisions.

Using a secure username and password, patients can view a broad array of health information, including physician visits, medications, immunizations, allergies, lab results, discharge summaries and other pertinent information in their personal record. Patients can also exchange secure, preferably encrypted, emails with their care teams, request prescription refills, schedule appointments for clinic visits or diagnostic tests, review coverage and benefits, update demographic information, download forms, make payments and access educational materials.

A well-designed patient portal improves efficiency and productivity between patients and providers. It can significantly enhance patient-provider communication and support care between visits. Most importantly, a growing number of studies have demonstrated that patient portals can improve patient outcomes. For example, Kaiser Permanente demonstrated that their patient portal improved medication adherence and resulted in lowered LDL cholesterol in patients with diabetes.[122] This study's results, and the results of others like it, have broad implications for millions of patients who are expected to use patient portals that will roll out as a part of Stage 2 Meaningful Use criteria.

The major disadvantage of most patient portals is that they link to a single healthcare provider. If a patient uses more than one healthcare organization (a common scenario), the patient needs to log on to each organization's portal to access their information and interact with the system. This results in a fragmented view of their health information and a disjointed flow of care delivery. These interoperability issues need to be addressed.

Over time, patient portals will likely evolve to support electronic visits, so-called e-visits. While e-visits offer advantages to any patient, they particularly benefit patients who live in remote rural areas. A visit via the Internet is often less expensive and more convenient than traveling a great distance for care, particularly when the patient only has questions, simple requests or minor medical complaints. Currently, few insurers reimburse for e-visits, but this is starting to change because of the potential for e-visits to lower the costs of care delivery.

> "Over time, patient portals will likely evolve to support electronic visits, so-called e-visits. While e-visits offer advantages to any patient, they particularly benefit patients who live in remote rural areas."

More sophisticated, next-generation portals will likely offer even more features, including more effective health information exchange, interoperability, data analytics and population health management. Patient-reported health, disease and outcome information from patient portals will provide considerably more data for health systems to use as they strive to improve outcomes and the health and well-being of the populations of patients they serve.

The evolving role of social media in healthcare

While social networking has probably been around for as long as humans have existed, recent technology advances have greatly facilitated the ability of people to connect anytime and anywhere in the world. Internet-based social networking services provide a platform for building networks and relationships among people who share common interests, activities, backgrounds, acquaintances and life situations. The typical social networking service provides participants an opportunity to share their personal profile, interests, social links, needs and opinions. In addition to providing users a web-based public or private profile, the service can create and share lists of connections and view cross-connections within the networking system.

Examples of modern web-based social networks include Facebook, Google+, LinkedIn, Instagram, Pinterest, Tumblr, Twitter and YouTube. These services provide tools that allow participants to interact via the Internet using a variety of methods, including posting, email and instant messaging. These tools facilitate mobile connectivity, media sharing (e.g., photos, videos, audio and events) and the sharing of ideas and interests. Social networking sites are increasingly becoming real time, allowing people the opportunity to instantly share ideas and opinions as situations evolve. Twitter is an excellent example of this trend, though not the only one.

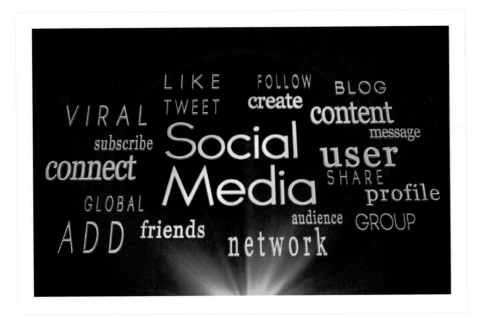

Organizations have begun to merge their business strategies and needs with social networking and cloud computing. Using these tools, companies can connect people based on shared business needs and experiences. In some cases, companies accomplish this via their own websites, and in other instances, they use an established social networking site like Facebook, LinkedIn or Twitter.

Social networking sites have experienced explosive growth. A recent Pew survey demonstrated that as of May 2013, 72 percent of online adults use social networking sites. Young adults are the most likely to say they use social media sites, while women and urban residents are more likely than men and rural dwellers to use these tools.[123]

Healthcare has been slow to embrace information technologies, but this is rapidly changing. Stimulated by the Health Information Technology for Economic and Clinical Health (HITECH) Act, EHRs and other IT systems are becoming more commonplace in healthcare. Social media tools are also establishing a presence in healthcare and transforming it in the process. The potential for social networking to improve communication, empower patients and enhance quality has been reviewed in several studies.[124, 125, 126]

The quantity of information that people seek and share online is staggering. For example, Google can access almost every online resource in the world. In 2013, Google managed almost 12.5 billion searches a month.[127] As of January 2014, Facebook had 180 million users in the U.S. alone and 1.3 billion users worldwide.[128] As of late 2013, Twitter had approximately 1 billion users worldwide, had supported roughly 300 billion Tweets, and their rate of Tweets per day had grown to 500 million.[129] The amount of information available on these sites about people and their preferences is truly amazing.

Social network sites like Facebook and Twitter develop insights by analyzing information about their users to understand their interests, beliefs and needs. They use the information to improve the user experience and to support their commercial success. Businesses worldwide are also starting to explore the potential of social media analytics for strategic advantage. These organizations are beginning to understand the vast intelligence that can be derived by looking at millions of conversations taking place on a routine basis, generally out in the open, between people who engage in social media.

Social media analytics requires tools that can handle the massive complexity, scale, speed and computation requirements associated with enormous data sets characteristic of social media in a way that is also cost effective. These requirements strain traditional analytical tools and require new approaches, as described below.

Social media and social media analytics offers enormous opportunities in healthcare. The Internet is widely accepted as a go-to source for consumers searching for healthcare information. Health research has consistently been one of the top web-based activities. However, consumers are not just doing online searches for health information. They are engaging in two-way communication with healthcare providers and other patients regarding health issues. When done well, social media analytics presents an entirely new world of opportunity for healthcare providers, insurers and policymakers. It can be a powerful tool for improving care delivery; enhancing patient, provider and population communications; and reducing costs.

> "When done well, social media analytics presents an entirely new world of opportunity for healthcare providers, insurers and policymakers. It can be a powerful tool for improving care delivery; enhancing patient, provider and population communications; and reducing costs."

As healthcare moves to a more value-based, outcomes-based system, healthcare providers must address several needs that are impacted by social media:

- Improved quality of care. Health systems increasingly need to eliminate medication errors and improve treatment compliance, improve communications and effectively educate patients and populations, especially those with chronic diseases. Social media offers the potential for a more effective and efficient way to share best practices and to collaborate with patients on treatment and innovation.

- Enhanced understanding and management of trends. Social media analytics offers healthcare providers an opportunity to better understand trends in attitudes, health, disease, compliance, needs and market forces.

- Reduced costs. Healthcare providers will use social media tools to more efficiently communicate with and educate the patients and populations they serve. These networks can also be used to help patients make better health-related decisions.

- ⊙ **Increased market share.** In an increasingly competitive environment, health systems need to more effectively personalize care, enhance patient experiences and control costs. As in other industries, social media tools and analytics can be very effective in addressing important market needs.

- ⊙ **Chronic disease management.** Heart disease, hypertension, diabetes, cancer and other chronic conditions are leading causes of death and disability, yet they are often not efficiently and effectively treated. Healthcare providers can use social media to identify ways to prevent and manage these conditions more efficiently, thereby lowering costs. Managing chronic conditions accounts for approximately 75 percent of U.S. healthcare expenditures. Anything that allows this treatment to be more efficient reduces costs.

The geometric growth in mobile devices and social media leaves healthcare providers in a better position to improve care, lower costs and contend with an increasingly competitive environment. To do so, they will need to become adept at complex social media analytics.

Realizing the promise of telehealth

Telehealth refers to the use of electronic information and telecommunications technologies to support remote clinical care, patient and professional education, public health and health administration. Telehealth connects care providers and patients through online encounters that are often as good as in-person visits, yet they are less expensive and more convenient for both patients and care providers.

There are a growing number of successful telehealth programs across the United States:

- ⊙ The Veterans Administration Care Coordination Home Telehealth program has shown that telehealth can be deployed and managed on a very broad scale while achieving cost-effective, high-quality outcomes for chronic care patients.

- ⊙ Partners Healthcare's Connected Cardiac Care Program for heart failure patients has generated an estimated $10 million in savings since 2006 for more than 1,200 enrollees.

- ⊙ Colorado-based Centura Health at Home has merged a clinical call center with telehealth to improve outcomes in elderly patients after discharge from the hospital.

The Commonwealth Fund has studied each of these telehealth examples and published case studies about them.[130]

The largest randomized, controlled trial of telehealth in the world is the United Kingdom's Department of Health's Whole System Demonstrator project.[131] The study was launched in May 2008 and involves 6,191 patients and 238 family physician practices across three communities in the UK: Newham, Kent and Cornwall. Three thousand and thirty people with one of three conditions — diabetes, heart failure (HF) or chronic obstructive pulmonary disease (COPD) — were included in the telehealth trial. Results published to date include:

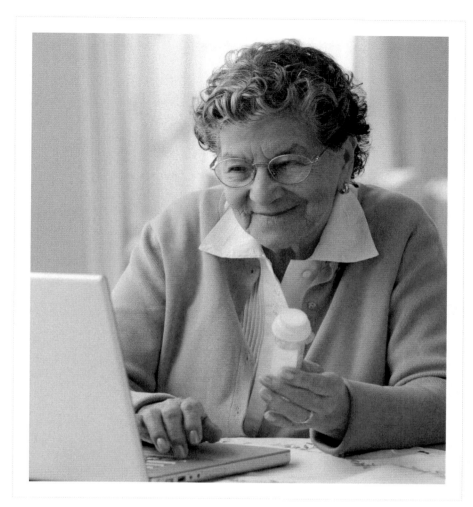

- 45 percent reduction in mortality rates

- 20 percent reduction in emergency admissions

- 15 percent reduction in clinic visits

- 14 percent reduction in elective admissions

- 14 percent reduction in bed days

Technologies used in telehealth include videoconferencing, the Internet, imaging, streaming media and land-based or wireless communications. While the technologies required to support telehealth services are readily available today, widespread adoption remains fairly low because of a variety of reimbursement, financial, interoperability, legal and policy barriers.

Similar to patient portals and social media, telehealth promises to efficiently extend the reach of healthcare providers, improve outcomes and provide rich new sources of data regarding patient populations for analysis. The IOM has published a detailed review of telehealth and its role in the evolving healthcare environment.[132]

The potential of remote patient monitoring

Remote patient monitoring (RPM) refers to using digital technology of different types to monitor patients outside of traditional clinical settings like the clinic, ED or hospital. This type of monitoring often occurs in the home, but with the advent of powerful mobile technologies like smartphones and the widespread availability of the Internet and cellular networks, monitoring can occur almost anywhere.

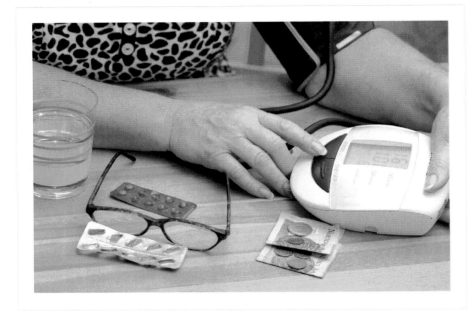

RPM uses digital sensors to collect a wide variety of data: physiologic data (blood pressure, weight, glucose levels, oxygen saturation, respiratory rate, tidal volume, etc.), fall data, nutrition information and medication administration data, to name a few. Digital devices can be scales, blood pressure cuffs, pulse oximeters, glucometers, fall sensors, drug dispensing devices and a host of other sensors that support a wide variety of functions. Once data is collected, it is transmitted to care provider organizations over the Internet. Because these technologies are mobile, they can support monitoring and care continuously, 24 hours a day, in any location. These devices can monitor patients, particularly those with chronic diseases, more carefully and continuously, increasing the likelihood that patient deterioration can be identified early so care can be more proactive.

These sensors can also have educational and decision support capabilities. For example, they can advise patients when to take medications, when to contact their provider team or when to seek medical attention in the clinic or hospital.

Most RPM technologies follow a general architecture that consists of five key components:

⊙ Monitoring sensors built into or connected to a device that supports wireless communications.

⊙ Local storage at the patient's site (often a home PC, tablet or smartphone) that provides an interface between the monitoring device and a centralized data repository, usually located at a healthcare provider institution.

- An Internet or cellular wireless connection.

- A centralized repository, generally located at a provider site, to store data sent from sensors, local storage devices and diagnostic applications.

- Diagnostic application software, frequently expert ruled-based, that identifies patients who need attention and often generates intervention alerts or treatment recommendations.

There are many published studies demonstrating how RPM sensors can improve outcomes and reduce costs, especially for chronic disease populations. This is not surprising since these devices offer the potential of more quickly identifying patients who are deteriorating, allowing provider resources to focus attention on those who most need care. Some studies have suggested that the cost of managing some of the most common chronic conditions could be lowered by up to 35-40 percent on an annualized basis using RPM.[133, 134, 135]

> "Once they are widely adopted, RPM technologies will result in massive streams of clinical data flowing back to healthcare organizations. Not only must this information become a logical part of a patient's electronic medical record, but advanced analytical capabilities will also be required to effectively manage and use the data."

Once they are widely adopted, RPM technologies will result in massive streams of clinical data flowing back to healthcare organizations. Not only must this information become a logical part of a patient's electronic medical record, but advanced analytical capabilities will also be required to effectively manage and use the data.

Genomics fuels personalized and predictive medicine

Genomics involves the study of a person's genes (the genome), including interactions between genes and in response to the person's environment. Genomes are the complete set of DNA within a single organism. Genomics applies DNA sequencing, recombinant DNA and bioinformatics to sequence, assemble and analyze the structure and function of genomes. Genomics also includes the scientific study of complex diseases — such as heart disease, asthma, diabetes and cancer — that are more typically caused by a combination of genetic and environmental factors than by individual genes alone.[136]

Genomics is helping researchers discover why some people get sick from certain infections, environmental factors and behaviors while others do not. For example, some people exercise their whole lives, eat a healthy diet, have regular medical checkups and die of a heart attack at age 40. Genomics also offers new possibilities for therapies and treatments for some complex diseases, as well as new diagnostic methods.

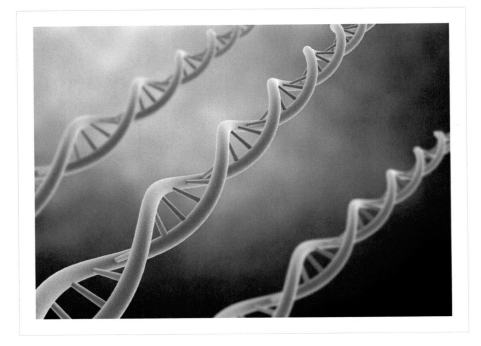

Genetic testing provides genetic information regarding vulnerabilities to inherited diseases and helps individuals and families learn how conditions such as sickle cell anemia and cystic fibrosis are inherited in families, what screening and testing options are available, and, for some genetic conditions, what treatments are available.

Next-generation genomic approaches and technologies promise clinicians and biomedical researchers the ability to drastically increase the amount of genomic data collected from large populations. Combining this with new informatics approaches that integrate many kinds of data with genomic data in disease research will permit researchers to better understand the genetic basis of drug responses and disease states.[137]

While medicine has always been inherently personal, the application of genomics to modern medicine enables a level of personalization that has not been previously possible or practical. Personal genomics is a powerful foundation for truly predictive medicine that draws on a patient's genetic profile to better understand their likelihood to develop disease as well as their response to both disease and treatment. By combining sequenced genomic data with other medical data, physicians will get a better understanding of an individual patient's potential for disease. This could lead to an era of personalized treatments for patients with a given disease, rather than the one-size-fits-all treatments of today. For this reason, some researchers in the field refer to the emergence of genomics as the era of personalized (or predictive) medicine.[138]

> " While medicine has always been inherently personal, the application of genomics to modern medicine enables a level of personalization that has not been previously possible or practical. "

The amount of data that has been and will be produced by sequencing, mapping and analyzing genomes will comfortably propel genomics and healthcare into the realm of "big data." Genomics produces huge volumes of data. Each human genome has 20,000-25,000 genes comprising over 3 billion base pairs. This amounts to 100,000 gigabytes of data. Sequencing many human genomes would quickly add up to hundreds of petabytes of data (a petabyte is 10^{15} bytes of digital information), and the data created by analysis of gene interactions multiplies the volumes of data even more.[139, 140]

Big data analytics — the next frontier for innovation, productivity, and health

The amount of data available in the world is growing exponentially, and analyzing large data sets — so-called big data — will become key for market analysis and competition, supporting new waves of productivity growth, innovation and consumer benefit. The increasing volume and detail of information captured by organizations — coupled with the rise of multimedia, social media and the Internet of Things (i.e., ubiquitous Internet-connected, data-collecting digital devices) — will fuel exponential growth in available data for many years ahead.

Big data has become a popular term to describe a massive volume of both structured and unstructured data that is so large it is difficult or impossible to process using traditional analytical methods and tools. In most situations, big data sets are so big, or change so fast, they exceed historical processing capacity. As of 2012, limits to the size of data sets that are possible to process in a reasonable amount of time were in the order of exabytes (a unit of information equal to one quintillion, 10^{18} bytes) of data.[141] Researchers routinely encounter limitations due to large data sets in genomics, meteorology, physics and biological and environmental research. These limitations are also increasingly being encountered in business, economics, finance and Internet searches. Increasingly ubiquitous information-gathering mobile devices, remote sensors, radio frequency identification (RFID) readers and wireless sensing networks are further exacerbating the volume of accessible data. As of 2012, the world was creating 2.5 exabytes of data every day.[142]

At what point something is called big data depends on the situation and the organization's capability to manage the data set. In some situations, hundreds of gigabytes of data may require more sophisticated analytical hardware and software tools, while in other instances it may take hundreds of terabytes before data size reaches this point.[143]

Given its present state, healthcare analytics pales in comparison to analytics performed in a number of scientific fields or by organizations such as Google, Facebook and others. However, with the advent of ACOs, patient portals, social media, medical homes, telehealth, remote patient monitoring and genomics, the volume of healthcare data at the disposal of healthcare providers will certainly grow exponentially in the years ahead, as will the need to glean information from this data to optimally manage population health. As healthcare systems steadily evolve into more sophisticated complex adaptive systems, these trends will definitely propel healthcare into the realm of big data.

There is no doubt that big data will generate value in healthcare. McKinsey & Company estimated that if U.S. healthcare were to use big data creatively and effectively to drive efficiency and quality, the healthcare sector could create more than $300 billion in value every year. Two-thirds of that would be in the form of reducing U.S healthcare expenditure by about 8 percent.[144] Realizing this goal will require all healthcare organizations to effectively implement the analytical infrastructure and improvement capabilities outlined in part 2 of this book (i.e., the three systems).

According to the International Institute of Analytics, there are a number of ways that analytics are likely to evolve over the next few years:[145]

- ⊘ Businesses will become increasingly reliant on analytics, and analytics will steadily become a key component of decision making and operations.

- ⊘ Traditional analytics will increasingly merge with big data analytics concepts and methods.

- ⊘ Currently, 95 percent of analytic capabilities are based in either reporting or visualizations. In the future, reporting will become more of an automated commodity (i.e., "self-service analytics"), and approximately 90 percent of analytic capabilities will shift toward predictive and prescriptive practices. Predictive analytics refers to the extraction of information from existing data sets with the goal of determining patterns in the data and predicting future outcomes and trends from the information. Predictive analytics cannot tell you exactly what will happen in the future, but it can forecast what might happen with an acceptable level of accuracy.[146]

- ⊘ As business intelligence tools improve, there will be more ability for front-line workers to manage data on their own to improve outcomes.

- ⊘ The role and size of enterprise analytics teams will grow, and more IT leaders will assume the role of "chief analytics officer."

- ⊘ Hadoop and other data frameworks will lead to earlier-stage data discovery by streamlining the extraction and analytic process. Apache's Hadoop (named after a toy elephant belonging to a co-creator's child) is an open source software framework for storage and large-scale processing of large data sets on clusters of commercially available hardware. The world's top search engines (Google, Yahoo, Facebook, etc.) use it because it makes it easier and cheaper to analyze and access the unprecedented volumes of data churned out by the Internet.[147] The enterprise data warehouse will continue to be essential, but over time, additional organizations and industries — including healthcare — are likely to use the Hadoop framework as they begin to wrestle with the challenges of big data.

- As data becomes more valuable as a competitive tool, organizations of all types will seek ways of monetizing information with varying degrees of success.

This is our opportunity — it is our revolution

This concludes our discussion of healthcare transformation. I hope, like me, that your passion and excitement for transformation has increased, and that you have learned the valuable role that you, as a clinician or healthcare leader, have in improving population outcomes, improving patients' experience and reducing costs.

This book was written with one goal in mind: to provide a credible and useful resource for those at the center of changing healthcare over the next few years. Based on my 43 years of experience, I know that individuals and organizations that implement the analytic, deployment and content systems discussed in chapters 3-6 will have a solid foundation from which to address healthcare needs today and in the future. As I mentioned in the introduction, this book is designed to be a dynamic resource. While it may find its way into print, it will remain primarily in digital format. As time and new experience leads to new knowledge, the book will be updated and improved so it can remain a valuable resource for driving meaningful change in healthcare.

There is no doubt that we live in interesting times. While challenging, healthcare transformation also promises to be exciting and rewarding for healthcare providers of all types, especially those who see beyond the challenges and appreciate a new future. How we view our present situation is up to us. One person's anxiety can be another person's opportunity. No doubt, creating a new future for healthcare will require time, effort, expertise, reliable data and analytics. However, the most important ingredient for change will be capturing the hearts and minds of healthcare's dedicated smart cogs, the clinicians who care for patients on a daily basis. Winning their allegiance is both possible and necessary.

The real question is, will we make history or become history? Those of us in healthcare today own the answer to this question. Creating a system of care that is better for those we serve is a noble endeavor. We need to leverage the incredible progress of the past century and design a new system that is more

> " The real question is, will we make history or become history? Those of us in healthcare today own the answer to this question. Creating a system of care that is better for those we serve is a noble endeavor. "

effective, more efficient and more capable of creating optimal outcomes for patients and communities. We need to move beyond the current widespread skepticism, frustration and fear to an era characterized by hope, excitement and promise. We have the necessary skills and technology solutions. The only real question is whether we have the will.

To paraphrase Sir William Osler's quote from the introduction to this book, we have an opportunity to witness a new birth of science, a new dispensation of health, a remodeled health system and a new outlook for humanity. Indeed, this is not an opportunity given to every generation. But it has been given to us. It is our revolution.

AUTHOR AND CONTRIBUTING EDITORS

Author

John Haughom, MD, Senior Advisor, Health Catalyst

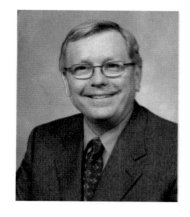

Dr. John Haughom is a healthcare executive with proven expertise in technology-enabled innovation, development of results-oriented strategic plans, leading multifaceted organization-wide change and directing complex operations. He has a proven record of turning vision into effective strategies and successfully implementing initiatives resulting in value including higher quality and safer care at the lowest possible cost. His broad knowledge of healthcare and emerging healthcare technologies is coupled with his recognized leadership abilities. Dr. Haughom's passion is engaging peer clinicians in creating the new era in healthcare, an era that holds great promise for the patients we serve.

Contributing editors

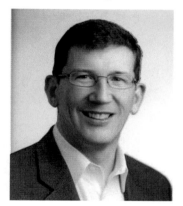

Thomas D. Burton, Co-Founder and Senior Vice President of Product Development, Health Catalyst

Mr. Burton is a co-founder of Health Catalyst and former President of the company. He brings 14 years of process improvement and IT experience to the company. Mr. Burton was a member of the team that led Intermountain Healthcare's nationally recognized improvements in quality of care delivery and reductions in cost. He has taught courses in the Advanced Training Program at Intermountain's Institute for Healthcare Delivery Research. Mr. Burton holds an MBA and a BS in Computer Science from Brigham Young University (BYU).

Holly Rimmasch, RN, Chief Clinical Officer, Health Catalyst

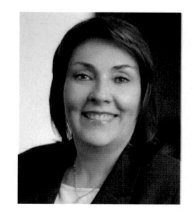

Ms. Rimmasch has over 28 years of experience in bedside care, as well as clinical and operational healthcare management. She has spent the last 17 years dedicated to improving clinical care, including implementation of operational best practices. Prior to joining Health Catalyst, Ms. Rimmasch was an Assistant Vice President at Intermountain responsible for Clinical Services and was integral in promoting integration of Clinical Operations across hospitals, ambulatory settings and managed care plans. Prior to her role in Clinical Services, she served as the Clinical Operations Director and Vice-Chair of Intermountain's Cardiovascular and Intensive Medicine Clinical Programs. Ms. Rimmasch holds a Master of Science in Adult Physiology from the University of Utah and a Bachelor of Science in Nursing from BYU.

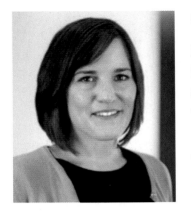

Cherbon VanEtten, Director of Education, Health Catalyst

Ms. VanEtten has 16 years of healthcare experience in information technology and healthcare analytics. Prior to joining Health Catalyst, she worked for MultiCare Health System as a senior project manager where she led numerous enterprise wide strategic initiatives — including the implementation of a healthcare data warehouse and quality improvement programs. She developed tools and methodologies to calculate ROI and total cost of ownership for IT investments – including EHR and EDW systems. Ms. VanEtten was responsible for leading a multidisciplinary clinical team in developing content for computerized physician order entry (CPOE), physician note templates and interdisciplinary plans of care. She earned her under graduate degree in Psychology from the University of Washington and a graduate degree in Biomedical Informatics from Oregon Health and Science University.

Dale Sanders, Senior Vice President, Health Catalyst

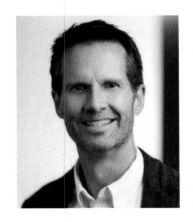

Prior to his work in the healthcare industry, Dale Sanders worked for 14 years in the military, national intelligence and manufacturing sectors, specializing in analytics and decision support. In addition to his role at Health Catalyst, Dale served as the senior technology advisor and CIO for the National Health System in the Cayman Islands. Previously, he was CIO of Northwestern University Medical Center and regional director of Medical Informatics at Intermountain, where he served in a number of capacities, including chief architect of Intermountain's enterprise data warehouse. He is a founder of the Healthcare Data Warehousing Association. He holds Bachelor of Science degrees in Chemistry and Biology from Fort Lewis College and is a graduate of the United States Air Force Information Systems Engineering Program.

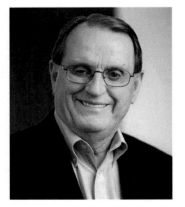

David Burton, MD, Executive Chairman, Health Catalyst

Dr. David A. Burton is executive chairman of Health Catalyst, which provides hospitals and health systems with Late-Binding™ data warehousing and healthcare analytics to transform clinical, financial and patient safety outcomes. A former Senior Vice President at Intermountain where he served a variety of executive positions over a period of 26 years, Dr. Burton spent the last 13 years of his career co-developing Intermountain's clinical process models utilized within the enterprise data warehouse environment. Dr. Burton is the former founding CEO of Intermountain's managed care plans (known as SelectHealth), which currently provide insurance coverage to approximately 500,000 members.

Leslie Falk, RN, MBA, PMP, Health Catalyst

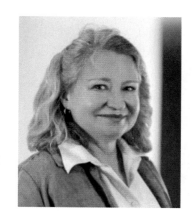

Prior to joining Health Catalyst, Leslie held positions as a Nurse Informaticist, Director of Biomedical Engineering, Clinical Engineer for Kaiser Permanente-Northern Region and Pediatric ICU RN. Ms. Falk also worked with Hewlett-Packard in several clinical, marketing, sales and support leadership roles. She holds a Master of Science degree in Community Counseling from Seattle Pacific University as well as an MBA and Bachelor of Science in Engineering from the University of Nevada, Las Vegas. Ms. Falk is also a certified Project Management Professional (PMP), Lean Green Belt and Information Privacy Professional (CIPP/CIPP IT).

Paul Horstmeier, Senior Vice President, Health Catalyst

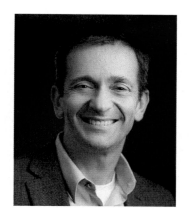

Mr. Horstmeier brings 25 years of Fortune 500 and small business operations and general management experience to Health Catalyst. He co-founded HB Ventures and filled senior executive roles at HB Ventures portfolio companies. Within Hewlett-Packard, Mr. Horstmeier launched and grew three different businesses, including co-founding HP's commercial e-commerce business which later expanded to include the management of the data systems and infrastructure for marketing operations across the company. As Vice President of HP.com, Paul headed up a 700-person organization that received nearly every industry award for quality and innovation during his tenure. Mr. Horstmeier holds an MBA and a BS in Computer Science from BYU.

Dan Burton, Chief Executive Officer, Health Catalyst

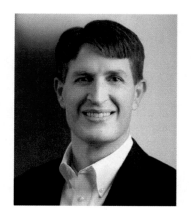

Dan Burton serves as CEO of Health Catalyst, a healthcare data warehousing and analytics company. He became involved with Health Catalyst when it was a three-person startup. Mr. Burton is also the co-founder of HB Ventures, the first investor in Health Catalyst. Prior to Health Catalyst and HB Ventures, Mr. Burton led the Corporate Strategy Group at Micron Technology (NASDAQ: MU). He also spent eight years with Hewlett-Packard (NYSE: HPQ) in strategy and marketing management roles. Before joining HP he was an associate consultant with the Boston Consulting Group, where he advised healthcare systems and technology companies. Mr. Burton holds an MBA with high distinction from Harvard University, where he was elected a George F. Baker Scholar, and a BS in economics, magna cum laude, from BYU.

REFERENCES

1.   US Department of Health and Human Services. *United States Life Tables. National Vital Statistics Reports.* 61(3); 1-63.

2.   Centers for Disease Control. Decline in deaths from heart disease and stroke — United States, 1900-1999. *JAMA.* 1999; 282(8): 724-6.

3.   US Department of Health and Human Services, Public Health Service. *Healthy People 2000: National Health Promotion and Disease Prevention Objectives.* Washington, DC: U.S. Government Printing Office. 1991. DHHS publication no. 91-50212.

4.   Wildavsky A. Doing better and feeling worse: the political pathology of health policy. *Daedelus.* 1977; 106(1): 105-123.

5.   McGinnis J, Williams-Russo P, Knickman JR. The case for more active policy attention to health promotion. *Health Affairs.* 2002; 21(2): 78-93.

6.   Khaw K, Wareham N, Bingham S, Welch A, Luben R, Day N. Combined impact of health behaviours and mortality in men and women: the EPIC Norfolk prospective population study. *PLoS Med.* 2008; (5): e12.

7.   Organization for Economic Cooperation and Development (OECD) Factbook 2013. OECD Web site. http://www.oecd-ilibrary.org/ economics/data/oecd-factbook-statistics/oecd-factbook-2013_data-00647-en. Published October 11, 2013. Accessed January 25, 2014.

8.   World health statistics 2009. World Health Organization (WHO) Web site.   http://www.who.int/whosis/whostat/EN_WHS09_Table7.pdf. Published 2009. Accessed January 25, 2014.

9.   Lalleman, NC. Reducing waste in health care. *Health Affairs Health Policy Brief.* December 13, 2012. http://www.healthaffairs.org/ healthpolicybriefs/brief.php?brief_id=82. Accessed January 25, 2014.

10.   Jonsen AR. Bentham in a box: Technology assessment and health care allocation. *Law Med Health Care.* 1986; 14(3-4): 172–174.

11.   Health at a glance 2011. Organization for Economic Cooperation and Development (OECD) Web site. http://www.oecd-ilibrary.org/social-issues-migration-health/health-at-a-glance-2011_health_glance-2011-en. Accessed January 25, 2014.

12.   Nolte E, McKee CM. In amenable mortality — deaths avoidable through health care — progress in the US lags that of three European countries. Health Affair [serial online]. 2012; 31(10): 2356.

13. Office of the Actuary, *National Health Expenditure Data.* Centers for Medicare and Medicaid Services, September 2007.

14. Hopson A, Retttenmaier A. Medicare spending across the map. National Center for Policy Analysis Web site. http://www.ncpa.org/pdfs/st313.pdf. Published July 2008. Accessed March 21, 2014.

15. Fisher E, et al. Health care spending, quality and outcomes. Dartmouth Institute for Health Policy and Clinical Practice Website. http://www.dartmouthatlas.org/downloads/reports/Spending_Brief_022709.pdf. Published February 2009. Accessed March 21, 2014.

16. Martin AB, et al. Growth in US health spending remained slow in 2010: health share gross domestic product was unchanged from 2009. *Health Affairs.* 2012; 31(1): 208-219.

17. Income, poverty and health insurance coverage in the United States: 2011. US Census Bureau Web site. http://www.census.gov/prod/2012pubs/p60-243.pdf. Published September, 2012. Accessed January 25, 2014.

18. Girod CS, Mayne LW, Weltz SA. 2012 Milliman medical index. McMillian Web site. http://www.milliman.com/insight/Periodicals/mmi/2012-Milliman-Medical-Index/. Published May 15, 2012. Accessed January 25, 2014.

19. Health security watch. Kaiser Family Foundation Web site. http://kff.org/health-costs/poll-finding/kaiser-health-security-watch/. Published June, 2012. Accessed January 25, 2014.

20. Committee on Quality in Health Care in America, Institute of Medicine. *Crossing the Quality Chasm: A New Health System for the 21st Century.* Washington, DC: National Academy Press; 2001.

21. Schuster MA, McGlynn EA, Brook RH. How good is the quality of healthcare in the United States? *Millbank Quarterly.* 1998; 76(4): 517-563.

22. McGlynn EA, Asch SM, Adams J, et al. The quality of health care delivered to adults in the United States. *NEJM.* 2003; 348(26): 2635-2645.

23. Donabedian, A. The quality of care: how can it be assessed? *JAMA.* 260(12): 1743-1748.

24. James BC. Quality improvement in health care: making it easy to do it right. *Journal of Managed Care Pharmacy.* 2002; 8(5): 394-397.

25. Protecting U.S. citizens from inappropriate medication use. Institute for Safe Medication Practice Web site. http://www.ismp.org/pressroom/

viewpoints/CommunityPharmacy.pdf. Published 2007. Accessed January 25, 2014.

26. Chassin M. Is health care ready for six sigma? *Millbank Quarterly.* 1998; 76(4): 565-591.

27. Fact sheet: The National Library of Medicine. US National Library of Medicine Web site. http://www.nlm.nih.gov/pubs/factsheets/nlm.html. Published October 26, 2012. Accessed January 25, 2014.

28. Shaneyfelt TM. Building Bridges to Quality. *JAMA.* 2001; 286(20): 2600-2601.

29. Williamson J, et al. *Medical practice information demonstration project: final report.* Office of the Asst. Secretary of Health, DHEW, Contract#282-77-0068GS. Baltimore, MD: Policy Research Inc., 1979.

30. Institute of Medicine. *Assessing Medical Technologies.* Washington, D.C.: National Academy Press; 1985.

31. Ferguson JH. Research on the delivery of medical care using hospital firms. Proceedings of a workshop. April 30 and May 1, 1990; Bethesda, Maryland. *Medical Care.* 1991; 29(7 Supplement): 1-2.

32. Eddy DM, Billings J. The quality of medical evidence: implications for quality of care. *Health Affairs.* 1988; 7(1): 19-32.

33. Kohn L, Corrigan J, Donaldson M, et al. *To err is human: building a safer health system.* Committee on Quality of Health Care in America, Institute of Medicine. Washington, DC: National Academy Press; 2000.

34. Wachter R. *Understanding Patient Safety* (Second edition). McGraw-Hill; 2012.

35. Hoyert DL, Arias E, Smith BL, Murphy SL, Kochanek KD. Deaths: final data for 1999. *National Vital Statistics Reports.* 2001; 49:8.

36. National Patient Safety Foundation. Agenda for Research and Development in Patient Safety. Chicago, IL: National Patient Safety Foundation. 2000.

37. Barach P, Small SD. Reporting and preventing medical mishaps: lessons from non-medical near miss reporting systems. *BMJ.* 2000; 320: 759-763.

38. Chassin MR, Galvin RW, and the National Roundtable on Health Care Quality. The urgent need to improve health care quality: Institute of Medicine national roundtable on health care quality. *JAMA.* 1998; 280: 1000-1005.

39. Mechanic D. Changing medical organizations and the erosion of trust. *Millbank Quarterly.* 1996; 74(2): 171-189.

40. Thomas EJ, Studdert DM, Burstin HR, et al. Incidents and types of adverse events and negligent care in Utah and Colorado. *Med Care.* 2000; 38: 261-271.

41. Turnbull JE, Mortimer J. *The business case for safety.* In: Zipperer LA and Cushman S, eds. Lessons in Patient Safety. Chicago, IL: National Patient Safety Foundation; 2001.

42. Wachter RM, Shojania KG. *Internal Bleeding: The Truth Behind America's Terrifying Epidemic of Medical Mistakes.* New York, NY: Rugged Land; 2004.

43. Wachter RM, Provonost PJ. Balancing "no blame" with accountability in patient safety. *NEJM.* 2009; 361: 1401-1406.

44. Kanjanarat P, Winterstein AG, Johns TE, et al. Nature of preventable adverse drug events in hospitals: a literature review. *American Journal Health Syst Pharm.* 2003; 60: 1750-1759.

45. Classen DC, Jaser L, Budnitz DS. Adverse drug events and potential adverse drug events among hospitalized Medicare patients: epidemiology and national estimates from a new approach to surveillance. *Joint Commission Journal of Quality and Patient Safety.* 2010; 36: 12-21.

46. *Preventing medication errors: A $21 billion opportunity.* Washington, DC; National Priorities Partnership and National Quality Forum; December 2010. www.qualityforum.org/NPP/docs/Preventing_Medication_Error_CAB.aspx. Accessed January 25, 2014.

47. Sarkar U, Wachter RM, Schroeder SA, et al. Refocusing the lens: patient safety in ambulatory chronic disease care. *Joint Commission Journal of Quality and Patient Safety.* 2009; 35: 377-383.

48. Gaba DM. Anesthesiology as a model for patient safety in health care. *BMJ.* 2000; 320: 785-788.

49. Thomas EJ, Studdert DM, Burstin HR, et al. Incidence and types of adverse events and negligent care in Utah and Colorado. *Med Care.* 2000; 38: 261-271.

50. Leape LL, Brennan TA, Laird N, et al. The nature of adverse events in hospitalized patients. Results of the Harvard Medical Practice Study II. *NEJM.* 1991; 324: 377-384.

51. Shojania KG. Changes in rates of autopsy-detected diagnostic errors over time: a systematic review. *JAMA.* 2003; 289: 2849-2856.

52. Lin L, Isla R, Doniz K, et al. Applying human factors to the design of medical equipment: patient controlled analgesia. *Journal Clin Monitor Computing.* 1998; 14: 253-263.

53. Zhang J, Johnson TR, Patel VL, et al. Using usability heuristics to evaluate patient safety of medical devices. *J Biomed Inform.* 2003; 36: 23-30.

54. Forster AJ, Murff HJ, Peterson JF, et al. The incidence and severity of adverse events affecting patients after discharge from the hospital. *Annals of Internal Medicine.* 2003; 138: 161-167.

55. Epstein AM. Revisiting readmissions — changing the incentives for shared accountability. *NEJM.* 2009; 360: 1457-1459.

56. Sexton JB, Thomas EJ, Helmreich RL. Error, stress, and teamwork in medicine and aviation: cross-sectional surveys. *BMJ.* 2000; 320: 745-749.

57. Statistical summary of commercial jet airplane accidents: Worldwide operations (1959-2012). Boeing Web site. http://www.boeing.com/news/techissues/pdf/statsum.pdf. Accessed January 25, 2014.

58. Sentinel event data: Root causes by event type (2004-2Q 2012). The Joint Commission Web site. http://www.jointcommission.org/assets/1/18/root_causes_event_type_2004_2Q2012.pdf. Accessed January 25, 2014.

59. Scott RD. The direct medical costs of healthcare-associated infections in U.S. hospitals and the benefits of prevention. Centers for Disease Control Web site. http://www.cdc.gov/hai/pdfs/hai/scott_costpaper.pdf. Published March 2009. Accessed January 25, 2014.

60. Pronovost PJ, et al. Sustaining reductions in catheter related bloodstream infections in Michigan intensive care units: observational study. *BMJ.* 2010; 340: c309.

61. Maziade PJ, Andriessen JA, Pereira P, et al. Impact of adding prophylactic probiotics to a bundle of standard preventative measures for Clostridium difficile infections: enhanced and sustained decrease in the incidence and severity of infection at a community hospital. *Curr Med Res Opin.* 2013; 29(10): 1341-7.

62. D'Amico R, et al. Antibiotic prophylaxis to reduce respiratory tract infections and mortality in adults receiving intensive care. The Cochrane Library 2009. http://onlinelibrary.wiley.com/doi/10.1002/14651858.CD000022.pub3/full. Accessed January 25, 2014.

63. Landrigan CP, Parry GJ, Bones CB, et al. Temporal trends in rates of patient harm resulting from medical care. *NEJM*. 2010; 363: 2124-2134.

64. Levinson DR. *Adverse events in hospitals: national incidence among Medicare beneficiaries*. Washington, DC: US Department of Health and Human Services, Office of the Inspector General; November 2010. Report No. OEI-06-09-00090.

65. Classen DC, Resar R, Griffin E, et al. 'Global Trigger Tool' shows that adverse events in hospitals may be ten times greater than previously measured. *Health Affairs*. 2011; 30: 581-589.

66. The healthcare imperative: lowering costs and improving outcomes: workshop series summary. The Institute of Medicine Web site. http://iom.edu/Reports/2011/The-Healthcare-Imperative-Lowering-Costs-and-Improving-Outcomes.aspx. Published February 24, 2011. Accessed February 1, 2014.

67. Health reform should focus on outcomes, not costs. Boston Consulting Group Web site. https://www.bcgperspectives.com/content/articles/health_care_payors_providors_health_reform_should_focus_on_outcomes/. Published October 30, 2012. Accessed February 1, 2014.

68. Taylor FW. *The Principles of Scientific Management*. New York, NY, USA and London, UK: Harper & Brothers; 1911.

69. Hastie T, Tibshirani, R, Friedman, J. *The Elements of Statistical Learning* (2nd edition). Springer; 2009.

70. Womack, JP, Roos, D, Jones, DT. *The Machine That Changed the World: The Story of Lean Production*. New York, NY: Harper Perennial; November 1991.

71. Going lean in health care. Institute for Healthcare (IHI) Innovation Series white paper. IHI Web site. http://www.ihi.org/resources/Pages/IHIWhitePapers/GoingLeaninHealthCare.aspx. Published 2005. Accessed February 1, 2014.

72. Morris ZS, Wooding S, Grant J. The answer is 17 years, what is the question: understanding time lags in translational research. *Journal of the Royal Society of Medicine* 2011; 104(12): 510-520.

73. Scherkenbach, WW. *The Deming Route to Quality and Productivity: Road Maps and Roadblocks*. Washington, DC: CEE Press Books, George Washington University; 1991.

74. Berwick DM, James B, Coye MJ. The connections between quality measurement and improvement. *Medical Care*. 2003; 41(1 Supplement): 30-38.

75. Shewhart, WA. *Economic control of quality of manufactured product.* New York, NY: D. Van Nostrand Company; 1931.

76. Schmittdiel JA, Grumbach K, Selby JV. System-based participatory research in health care: an approach for sustained translational research and quality improvement. *Annals of Family Medicine.* 2010; 8(3): 256-259.

77. Cleveland, WS. *The Elements of Graphing Data.* Summit, NJ: Hobart Press; 1994.

78. Tufte, ER. *The Visual Display of Quantitative Information.* Cheshire, CT: Graphics Press; 1990.

79. Tufte, ER. *Visual Explanations: Images and Quantities.* Cheshire, CT: Graphics Press; 1998.

80. Tufte, ER. *Evidence and Narration.* Cheshire, CT: Graphics Press; 1997.

81. Berwick DM. Controlling variation in health care: a consultation from Walter Shewhart. *Medical Care.* 1991; 29(12): 1212-25.

82. Readiness assessment & developing project aims. Health Resources and Services Administration. Department of Health and Human Services Web site. http://www.hrsa.gov/quality/toolbox/methodology/readinessassessment/. Accessed February 1, 2014.

83. Agency for Health Research and Quality (AHRQ) quality indicators toolkit. AHRQ Web site. http://www.ahrq.gov/professionals/systems/hospital/qitoolkit/a3-selfassessment.pdf. Accessed February 1, 2014.

84. Senge, Peter M. *The Fifth Discipline.* New York and Toronto: Doubleday/Currency; 1990.

85. Garvin DA, Edmondson AC, Gino F. Is yours a learning organization? *Harvard Business Review.* 2008; 86(3): 109-116.

86. McHugh D, Groves D, Alker, A. 1998. Managing learning: what do we learn from a learning organization? *The Learning Organization.* 1998; 5(5): 209-220.

87. Pedler M, Burgogyne J, Boydell, T. *The Learning Company: A strategy for sustainable development* (2nd edition). London: McGraw-Hill; 1997.

88. Institute of Medicine Roundtable on Value and Science-driven Health Care. *The Learning Health System Series.* Washington, DC: National Academy Press; 2001.

89. Institute of Medicine. *Best Care at Lower Cost: The Path to Continuously Learning Health Care in America.* Washington, DC: National Academy Press; 2013.

90. Rogers, EM. *Diffusion of innovations* (5th edition). New York, NY: Free Press; 2003.

91. Sackett DL, Rosenberg WM, Gray JA, Haynes RB, Richardson WS. Evidence based medicine: what it is and what it isn't. *British Medical Journal.* 1996; 312(7023):71-2.

92. Sackett DL, Rosenberg WM. The need for evidence-based medicine. *J Royal Soc Med.* 1995; 88(11): 620-624.

93. Sackett DL, Straus SE, Richardson WS, Rosenberg W, Haynes RB. *Evidence-based medicine: how to practice and teach EBM* (2nd edition). Edinburgh & New York: Churchill Livingstone, 2000.

94. Committee on Comparative Effectiveness Research Prioritization, Institute of Medicine. *Comparative Effectiveness Research.* Washington, DC: National Academy Press; 2013.

95. Roland M and Torgerson DJ. Understanding controlled trials: what are pragmatic trials? *BMJ.* 1998; 316: 285.

96. Grade definitions. United States Preventive Services Task Force Web site. http://www.uspreventiveservicestaskforce.org/uspstf/grades.htm. Accessed February 1, 2014.

97. Oxford Centre for Evidence-Based Medicine — levels of evidence and grades of recommendation. Centre for Evidence Based Medicine Web site. http://www.cebm.net/?o=1025. Published March 2009. Accessed February 1, 2014.

98. Lynn J, et al. The ethics of using quality improvement methods in health care. *Ann Intern Med.* 2007; 146: 666-674.

99. United States Department of Health and Human Services. Code of Federal Regulations 45CFR46.102. Department of Health and Human Services Web site: http://www.hhs.gov/ohrp/policy/ohrpregulations.pdf. Accessed February 1, 2014.

100. Andersen CA, Daigh RD. Quality mind-set overcomes barriers to success. *Healthcare Financial Management.* 1991; 45(2): 20-22.

101. James B, Bayley K. Cost of poor quality or waste in integrated delivery system settings. AHRQ Web site. http://www.ahrq.gov/research/findings/final-reports/costpqids/costpoorids.pdf. Published 2006. Accessed February 1, 2014.

102. Elective induction of labor: safety and harms. AHRQ Web site. http://effectivehealthcare.ahrq.gov/ehc/products/135/354/induction%20of%20labor%20clinician%20guide.pdf. Published 2009. Accessed March 12, 2014.

103. Caughey AB, et al., *Maternal and neonatal outcomes of elective induction of labor: a systematic review and cost-effectiveness analysis.* AHRQ. March 2009.

104. Eddy DM. Evidence-based medicine: a unified approach, *Health Affairs.* 2005; 24(1): 9-17.

105. Kindig D, Stoddart G. What is population health? *American Journal of Public Health.* 2003; 93(3): 380-383.

106. Meeting Report of World Conference of Social Determinants of Health held in Rio de Janeiro. WHO Web site. http://www.who.int/sdhconference/resources/Conference_Report.pdf. Published 2008. Accessed March 12, 2014.

107. McGinnis JM, Williams-Russo P, Knickman JR. 2002. The case for more active policy attention to health promotion. *Health Affairs.* 2002; 21(2): 78–93.

108. Frankish CJ, et al. *Health impact assessment tool for population health promotion and public policy.* Vancouver: Institute of Health Promotion Research, University of British Columbia, 1996.

109. World Health Organization. *WHO definition of health, preamble to the constitution of the World Health Organization* as adopted by the International Health Conference. New York, 1946.

110. World Health Organization. *Constitution of the World Health Organization – basic documents,* Forty-fifth edition, Supplement, October 2006.

111. Lee TH. Putting the value framework to work. *NEJM.* 2010; 363: 2481-2483.

112. Cox, T. Exposing the true risks of capitation financed healthcare. *Journal of Healthcare Risk Management.* 2011; 30: 34–41.

113. Flareau B, Bohn J, Konschak C. *Accountable Care Organizations: A Roadmap to Success.* Convurgent Publishing, LLC; 2011.

114. Bard M, Nugent M. *Accountable Care Organizations: Your Guide to Strategy, Design, and Implementation.* Health Administration Press; 2011.

115. Patient-centered Primary Care Collaborative. Joint Principles of the Patient-centered Medical Home. Patient Centered Primary Care Collaborative Web site. http://www.aafp.org/dam/AAFP/documents/practice_management/pcmh/initiatives/PCMHJoint.pdf. Published February, 2007. Accessed March 15, 2014.

116. Allred NJ, Wooten KG, Kong Y. The association of health insurance and continuous primary care in the medical home on vaccination coverage for 19- to 35-month-old children. *Pediatrics.* 2007; 119(S1): S4–11.

117. Schoen C, Osborn R, Doty MM, Bishop M, Peugh J, Murukutla N. Toward higher-performance health systems: adults' health care experiences in seven countries. *Health Affairs.* 2007; 26(6): 717–34.

118. Homer CJ, Klatka K, Romm D, et al. A review of the evidence for the medical home for children with special health care needs. *Pediatrics.* 2008; 122(4): 922–37.

119. Strickland BB, Singh GK, Kogan MD, Mann MY, van Dyck PC, Newacheck PW. Access to the medical home: new findings from the 2005-2006 National Survey of Children with Special Health Care Needs. *Pediatrics.* 2009; 123(6): 996–1004.

120. Reid RJ, Coleman K, Johnson EA, et al. The group health medical home at year two: cost savings, higher patient satisfaction, and less burnout for providers. *Health Affairs.* 2010; 29(5): 835–43.

121. National Academy of Sciences. *Primary Care: America's Health in a New Era.* Washington, DC, 1996.

122. Sarkar U, et al. Use of the refill function through an online patient portal is associated with improved adherence to statins in an integrated delivery health system. *Medical Care.* 2014; 52(3): 194-201.

123. Social networking use. Pew Research Center Web site. http://www.pewresearch.org/data-trend/media-and-technology/social-networking-use/. Accessed March 17, 2014.

124. Hawn C. Take two aspirin and tweet me in the morning: how Twitter, Facebook, and other social media are reshaping health care. *Health Affairs.* 2014; 33(3): 361-368.

125. Sharma S, Kilian R. Health 2.0 — lessons learned: social networking with patients for health promotion. *Journal of Primary Care and Community Health.* 2014; 39(1): 181-190.

126. Timian A, Rupcic S, Kachnowski S, Luis P. Do patients "like" good care? Measuring quality via Facebook. *American Journal of Medical Quality.* 2013; 28: 358.

127. Smith, C. By the numbers: 33 amazing Google stats and facts. Digital Marketing Ramblings Web site. http://expandedramblings.com/index.php/by-the-numbers-a-gigantic-list-of-google-stats-and-facts. Published February 2, 2014. Accessed March 15, 2014.

128. 3 Million teens leave Facebook in 3 years: the 2014 Facebook demographic report. iSTRATEGYBLABS Web site. http://istrategylabs. com/2014/01/3-million-teens-leave-facebook-in-3-years-the-2014-facebook-demographic-report/. Published January 15, 2014. Accessed March 15, 2014.

129. Smith, C. By the numbers: 116 amazing Twitter statistics. Digital Marketing Ramblings Web site. http://expandedramblings.com/index. php/march-2013-by-the-numbers-a-few-amazing-twitter-stats/#. UycrdNzEKG8. Published February 5, 2014. Accessed: March 15, 2014.

130. The promise of telehealth. Commonwealth Fund Connection Web site. http://www.commonwealthfund.org/Newsletters/The-Commonwealth-Fund-Connection/2013/Feb/February-4-2013.aspx. Published February, 4, 2013. Accessed March 15, 2014.

131. Steventon A, et al. Effect of telehealth on use of secondary care and mortality: findings from the Whole System Demonstrator cluster randomized trial. *BMJ.* 2012; 344: 3874.

132. National Research Council. *The role of telehealth in an evolving health care environment: workshop summary.* Washington, DC: The National Academies Press, 2012.

133. Cherry JC, et al. Diabetes management program for an indigent population empowered by telemedicine technology. *Diabetes Technology & Therapeutics.* 2002; 4(6): 783-791.

134. Gendelman S, et al. Improving asthma outcomes and self-management behaviors of inner-city children: a randomized trial of the health buddy interactive device and an asthma diary. *Archives of Pediatrics & Adolescent Medicine.* 2002; 156(2): 114-120.

135. Meyer M, Kobb R, Ryan P. Virtually health: chronic disease management in the home. *Disease Management.* 2002; 5(2): 87-94.

136. A brief guide to genomics. National Human Genome Research Institute Web site. http://www.genome.gov/18016863. Published October 19, 2011. Accessed March 14, 2014.

137. Feero WG, Guttmacher A, O'Donnell CJ, Nabel, E. Genomic medicine: genomics of cardiovascular disease. *NEJM.* 2011; 365(22): 2098–109.

138. Jorgensen J, Winther H. The era of personalized medicine: 10 years later. *Personalized Medicine.* 2009; 6(4): 423-428.

139. High performance computing and data storage. New York Genome Center Web site. http://www.nygenome.org/genomics/high-performance-computing/. Accessed March 15, 2014.

140. International Human Genome Sequencing Consortium. Finishing euchromatic sequence of the human genome. *Nature.* 2004; 431(7011): 931–945.

141. Francis, M. Future telescope array drives development of exabyte processing. ARS Technica Web site. http://arstechnica.com/science/2012/04/future-telescope-array-drives-development-of-exabyte-processing/. Published April 2, 2012. Accessed March 15, 2014.

142. McAfee A, Brynjolfsson E. Big data: the management revolution. *Harvard Business Review.* 2012; 90(10): 60-69.

143. Guterman, J. Release 2.0: issue 11. O'Reilly Media; 2009. http://www.oreilly.com/data/free/release-2-issue-11.csp. Accessed March 1, 2014.

144. Manyika J, Chui M, Brown B, Bughin J, Dobbs R, Roxburgh C, Byers A. Big data: the next frontier for innovation, competition and productivity. McKinsey & Company Insights & Publications Web site. http://www.mckinsey.com/insights/business_technology/big_data_the_next_frontier_for_innovation. Published May 2011. Accessed March 15, 2014.

145. Davenport T. The rise of analytics 3.0: how to compete in the data economy. International Institute for Analytics Web site. http://info.iianalytics.com/a3-ebook. Published 2003. Accessed March 2, 2014.

146. Eckerson W. Predictive analytics: extending the value of your data warehousing investment. TDWI Web site. http://tdwi.org/articles/2007/05/10/predictive-analytics.aspx?sc_lang=en. Published May 10, 2007. Accessed March 3, 2014.

147. Vance A. Hadoop, a free software program, finds uses beyond search. New York Times. March 16, 2009. http://www.nytimes.com/2009/03/17/technology/business-computing/17cloud.html?_r=0. Accessed March 3, 2014.

148. Zimmerman B, Lindberg C, Plsek P. *Edgeware: Insights from Complexity Science for Health Care Leaders.* Irving, Texas: VHA Inc.; 1998.

149. Hoffman E. Women's health and complexity science. *Academic Medicine.* 2000; 75(11): 1102-1106.

150. "Applying Complexity Science to Health and Healthcare" in the *Plexus Institute Newsletter,* May 2003. Available at: http://c.ymcdn.com/sites/www.plexusinstitute.org/resource/collection/6528ED29-9907-4BC7-8D00-8DC907679FED/11261_Plexus_Summit_report_Health_Healthcare.pdf.

151. Miller GA. The magical number is seven, plus or minus two: Some limits on our capacity for processing information. *Psychological Review.* 1956; 63(2): 81-97.

152. East TD, Bohm SH, Wallace CJ, et al. A successful computerized protocol for clinical management of pressure control inverse ratio ventilation in ARDS patients. *Chest.* 1992; 101(3): 697-710. doi: 10.1378/chest.101.3.697.

153. Institute of Medicine. *Crossing the Quality Chasm: A New Health System for the 21st Century. Appendix B: Redesigning Health Care with Insights from the Science of Complex Adaptive Systems.* Washington, DC: National Academy Press; 2001.

154. Gawande A. *The Checklist Manifesto: How to Get Things Right.* New York, NY: Metropolitan Books; 2009.

155. Mick SM, Wyttenback, et al. *Advances in Health Care Organization Theory.* San Francisco, CA: Jossey-Bass; 2003.

156. Rouse WB. Health care as a complex adaptive system: Implications for design and management. *The Bridge.* 2008; 38(1); 17-25.

157. Wheeler DJ. *Understanding Variation: The Key to Managing Chaos (Second Edition).* Knoxville, TN: SPC Press; 2000.

158. Cary RG, Lloyd RC. *Measuring Quality Improvement in Healthcare: A Guide to Statistical Process Control Applications.* New York, NY: ASQ Quality Press; 2001.

159. Hart M, Hart RF. *Statistical Process Control for Healthcare.* Cengage Publishing; 2001.

APPENDIX A: HEALTHCARE: A COMPLEX ADAPTIVE SYSTEM

Defining complexity science

Complexity science is the study of complex adaptive systems, the relationships within them, how they are sustained, how they self-organize and the outcomes that result. Complexity science is made up of a variety of theories and concepts. It is a multidisciplinary field involving many different areas of study, including biology, mathematics, anthropology, economics, sociology, management theory, computer science and others.

Complexity science is built on modern research and concepts that view systems as nonlinear and able to adapt to a changing environment. Complexity science considers characteristics of systems that are overlooked by conventional mechanical approaches. It offers a framework for studying complex adaptive systems, focusing on the patterns and relationships among the parts in order to understand and act on the unpredictable aspects of working with people in dynamic organizations.[148, 149]

A complex adaptive system is a collection of individual entities that have the ability to act in ways that are not always totally predictable. Furthermore, the entities' actions are interconnected: one entity's actions can sometimes change the context for the other entities and thereby impact the other entities' actions in unpredictable ways. Examples of complex adaptive systems include the environment, the immune system, the stock market, a colony of insects, world financial markets and families.

Mechanical versus complex theories

For centuries, scientists viewed the world and events as being linear. Their world was one where simple cause-and-effect rules could generally explain events and outcomes. Everything was viewed as a machine. If you carefully took the machine apart and gained understanding of the parts, you could then understand the whole. Scientists embraced the belief that the universe and all of its components could be dissected, understood and ultimately controlled.

However, in the modern era, this view of the universe and its parts began to falter. Despite intensive study, many systems did not behave in this manner. The weather, ecosystems, economics, political systems and, increasingly, organizations as they became larger and more complex, could not be predicted by mechanical theory. Despite using the most powerful computers in the world, these types of systems, and others like them, remained unpredictable and hard to understand. Ultimately, as science entered the world of quantum physics, the reality that mechanical theory could not explain everything became more obvious. Increasingly, new discoveries made it apparent that the very smallest nuclear subcomponents simply did not behave in accordance with simple cause-and-effect rules. They were governed by a different set of principles.

As scientists in different disciplines explored these phenomena, a new theory began to emerge that better explained the behavior and outcomes of these complex systems: complexity theory. In a complex system, the system is made up of components that can act independently and interact in a way that is unpredictable. Yet these interactions, and the system as a whole, ultimately can be explained by complexity theory.

You can distinguish between systems that are fundamentally mechanical and those that are naturally adaptive. Conventional (mechanical) models are based on Newtonian scientific principles that view the universe and its subsystems as machines. In the Newtonian approach, theory holds that by understanding simple, universal rules that control the system's parts, future behavior of the parts is predictable with linear cause and effect. Even complex mechanical systems rarely produce unpredictable behavior. When they appear to, experts can generally sift through the data and determine the cause. For example, when a computer system crashes, it may appear that the outcome was unpredictable. However, more often than not, you can decipher the cause after a thoughtful and thorough review of the evidence. A reasonable argument can be made that this framework for understanding how machines work guided the orientation of medicine around organ-based disciplines and physiological processes and healthcare organizations around linear, hierarchal relationships and rules.

Conversely, the agents within a complex system interact and connect with each other in random ways. Complexity science helps make regularities become apparent, it helps form a pattern that feeds back into the system, and it informs the interactions of the agents within the system and the behavior of the system as a whole. For example, if an organism within an ecosystem begins to deplete one species, the result will be a greater or smaller supply of food for others in the system, which affects their behaviors and numbers. Following a period of flux across all the different populations within the ecosystem, a new balance or steady state emerges.

The growing interest in complexity theory

The interest in complexity science has grown rapidly over the past decade. One of the reasons for this is the emergence of highly complex, worldwide challenges, including the environment, understanding the human genome, healthcare and medicine, economics, world markets, population growth and telecommunications, to name a few. Another reason is the emergence of advanced computing resources with sufficient power to model large-scale, complex systems, to investigate new ways of approaching system design and to predict the outcomes for a given model. With advanced computing systems, experts are able to effectively study large-scale, complex, highly adaptive systems, like healthcare.

Organisms, people and organizations are parts of networks within complex adaptive groups. They interact, adapt and learn. For example, organisms are the adaptive agents within an ecosystem; antibodies are the adaptive agents in the immune system; humans are the adaptive agents in the political system; and organizations are the adaptive agents in the economic system. Each agent acts based on its knowledge and experience, and all agents interact together, while adapting to the environment. In complex adaptive systems, the parts have the freedom and ability to respond to stimuli in different and unpredictable ways. As a result, unpredictable, surprising and even innovative behaviors and outcomes become real possibilities.

Complexity theory and organizations

Although its roots are clearly in science, complexity theory is increasingly being used outside of science to help describe, understand and predict the behavior of other complex entities, including organizations. Complexity science can help you understand how an organization and its subcomponents adapt to their environments and how they cope with complexity and uncertainty. From the perspective of complexity science, organizations are not viewed as aggregations of individual static entities that behave in predictable ways.

Rather, they are viewed as a dynamic collection of strategies and structures that are adaptive. That is, their collective behavior will evolve and self-organize in response to change, initiating events or collections of events that can be explained by complexity science. By understanding the tenets of complexity science, leaders of complex organizations can better understand and lead their organizations. However, this requires leaders to view and lead their organizations differently than they have traditionally.

| Comparison of organizational system characteristics ||
Complex adaptive systems	Traditional systems
Are living organisms	Are machines
Are unpredictable	Are controlling and predictable
Are adaptive, flexible, creative	Are rigid, self-preserving
Tap creativity	Control behavior
Embrace complexity	Find comfort in control
Evolve continuously	Recycle

Figure 105: Comparison of organizational system characteristics

Comparison of leadership styles	
Complex adaptive systems	**Traditional systems**
Are open, responsive, catalytic	Are controlling, mechanistic
Offer alternatives	Repeat the past
Are collaborative, co-participating	Are in charge
Are connected	Are autonomous
Are adaptable	Are self-preserving
Acknowledge paradoxes	Resist change, bury contradictions
Are engaged, continuously emerging	Are disengaged, nothing ever changes
Value persons	Value position, structures
Shift as processes unfold	Hold formal position
Prune rules	Set rules
Help others	Make decisions
Are listeners	Are knowers

Figure 106: Comparison of leadership styles

Organizational management theorist Gareth Morgan, Ph.D., contrasted complex adaptive systems and traditional systems, as shown in Figure 105.[150] Change and innovation are major characteristics of complex adaptive systems, as opposed to the simple, linear and additive relations that are characteristic of Newtonian, mechanical thinking. Behaviors and outcomes can be good or bad, advances or failures. Outcomes can occur either at the microsystem level (for example, an outcome resulting from a relationship of trust between a patient and a physician) or at the macrosystem level of care (such as the AIDS epidemic).

Complexity science views individual organizations as part of a connected web of interacting agents embedded in larger networks and systems, distinct from traditional top-down, linear, prescriptive, bureaucratic hierarchies. Living in this world of organizational interconnections can create an uncontrollable and oftentimes turbulent environment. The consequences of people interacting in a complex organizational system (especially those with slim resources) can contribute to leaders feeling like they are living in a world of unpredictable disruptions, not a world of understandable trends. As they continue to operate in this context, leaders need to become more skilled in managing contradictions and competing demands. In Figure 106, Morgan contrasts the leadership styles necessary to lead in a complex adaptive system environment as compared to a traditional system.

Viewing healthcare as a complex adaptive system

As discussed in chapter 2, most people would agree that healthcare is overwhelmingly complex. In the 1960s, the typical general practitioner practiced in a privately owned office with minimal staff, subscribed to one or two journals, periodically engaged a specialist when necessary, rounded on their patients in the hospital and did roughly an hour's worth of paperwork a week. The specialist was completely independent, practiced primarily in the hospital, focused primarily on a particular body system, was in total control of their practice and interacted with administrators only when they needed some type of support (e.g., a new device).

Those days are essentially gone. As thousands of new drug therapies, sophisticated new forms of diagnosis and treatment, the need for computerization, demands for integrated care, rising demands for data-driven quality outcomes, increasing costs, growing legal liabilities, complex new regulations, and a host of other complex, interrelated forces entered the scene, the complexity of clinical care grew exponentially. With these changes, the practice of care has become stressful and often overwhelming for both clinicians and non-clinicians, from individual providers, nurses, general practitioners and specialists to administrators and senior executives.

As the healthcare environment becomes even more complex, it is increasingly exceeding the ability of the smartest and most well-trained clinician to consistently make the best possible decisions. Studies have shown that humans can deal with approximately seven (plus or minus two) independent variables when making any given decision, regardless of how smart or how well educated they are.[151] Yet clinicians encounter situations almost every day that require juggling far more than seven variables. For example, Alan Morris, MD, demonstrated that there are about 240 factors to consider when adjusting a ventilator for a patient in an intensive care unit.[152] Although Dr. Morris concluded that only about 40 of these were the most important, that number still vastly exceeds the ability of the unaided human mind.

Regardless of the clinical environment in which they practice, busy clinicians and health system leaders face multivariable, complex decisions every day. Given their human limitations, it is not surprising that they would find it difficult to consistently make the right decision. As healthcare becomes even more complex, it will be increasingly necessary to build standardized processes, care environments and decision-support systems that allow clinicians and others to be the best they can be.

In Appendix A of the IOM's Crossing the Quality Chasm report, *Redesigning Health Care With Insights From the Science of Complex Adaptive Systems*, Paul Plsek defined a system as "the coming together of parts, interconnections, and purpose."[153] While systems can be broken down into parts that can be individually interesting, the real power lies in the way the parts come together and are interconnected to fulfill a given purpose. The U.S. healthcare system is made up of numerous parts (hospitals, clinics, laboratories, pharmacies, urgent care centers, imaging centers, physician groups, insurers, etc.) that are interconnected by patients and the flow of information to fulfill a specific purpose — improving and maintaining the health of patients and populations.

It is easy to demonstrate that the U.S. healthcare system and its many stakeholders (patients, care providers, operational stakeholders, payers, policymakers, society, etc.) represent a complex adaptive system. While there are certainly pockets of mechanical systems within healthcare, the individual parts and the collective whole largely represents a complex adaptive system.

In his book *The Checklist Manifesto: How to Get Things Right*, Atul Gawande points out that complexity theory divides decisions and problems into three general categories: simple, complicated and complex.[154] Simple problems are ones in which the inputs and the outputs are known. These problems can be managed by following a set of rules. Complicated decisions involve significant uncertainty. In these situations, the solutions may not be known, but they are potentially knowable. Finally, complex decisions are decisions in which the actual formula for success is unknowable. You may have a general sense for what works, but you do not know with certainty what will work, nor do you know the outcome with any degree of certainty. Raising a child is a good example. You can raise children using the best available, experienced-based guidance, yet the outcome is definitely not predictable.

It is important to understand the differences between these three categories of decisions and problems because the approach you take needs to match the type of problem you face. For example, a surgical checklist or simple datasets have been proven to be good solutions for simple problems. However, a checklist or a simple dataset is unlikely to be of much help for a highly complex decision. The best approach to a complex decision is often to try something that seems to make sense based on your knowledge and the available data. You must then measure the results and often repeat the cycle many times in search of the best possible outcome. This data-driven approach is increasingly being used in clinical care and will be become even more common in the future.

Complexity science can guide your understanding of the healthcare system, a multilayered system driven largely by rapidly changing demands, technology and information. In healthcare, organization and practitioner components make up a continuously evolving system because of their innovative, diverse and progressive adaptations. Understanding the core processes of an organizational system is critical. Core processes are the building blocks of the organizational system.

Studying the interfaces and interactions of core processes allows health system leaders to ask questions based on flows and patterns among the processes, identify feedback loops, explore interfaces and interactions and ultimately recognize the elements of an efficient system. If the components of a complex adaptive system act collectively, broken healthcare system interconnections can be identified and changed. When interactions among these components encounter boundaries, those boundaries can constrain effective interactions and limit outcomes. For example, if the traditional silos that have characterized our healthcare system persist (e.g., physicians, hospitals, insurers, etc.), they will impede the development of efficient accountable care organizations that can effectively manage the health and wellbeing of populations.

Whether you look at population health management or individual patient care, the traditional approach to patient care delivery and health system leadership does not encompass the complexity and behavior of the whole system. In managing individual patient care, clinicians tend to pay attention to linear episodes of care, one organ or disease at a time. However, the body has multiple systems, and treatment directed to one organ system or disease potentially affects the entire body.

The same is true of health system leadership. Healthcare organizations tend to focus their resources on treating, restoring and maintaining their own system integrity. Like the human body system, the healthcare organization has multiple, interconnected components. Healthcare delivery organizations are complex organizational forms, and they operate in an environment that is among the most complex of the world's organizational environments. Hundreds of different types of professionals and organizations interact to provide a wide variety of services to patients, their families and their communities. Fragmentation and specialization, much of it well intended, characterizes both the delivery of health services and healthcare policy. We often fail to appreciate how these separate components interconnect. Similar to multiple organ failure in illness, failure of healthcare organizations to reach their potential often results from a failure to understand relationships and interactions between subcomponents. This can lead to significant dysfunction, or worse, the failure of the system. It also prevents the realization of optimal care for patients and communities.

Going forward, complexity science will play an increasing role in the design of new care delivery systems and models (at both the microsystem and macro-system level) and in the development of new policies designed to shape and transform our healthcare delivery system. Readers interested in learning more about viewing healthcare as a complex adaptive system and the application of complexity science to healthcare can access a variety of available resources.[20, 155, 156]

APPENDIX B: UNDERSTANDING DATA TYPES IN HEALTHCARE

In chapter 4, we covered the concept of processes and systems, the elements of frequency distributions, how to understand the different types of variation (common cause and assignable) and how they relate to processes. We also reviewed the concept of statistical process control and how it helps differentiate common cause variation from assignable variation, how statistical process control (SPC) charts are created, how SPC charts are applied and tampering. Professionals involved in healthcare improvement should understand these concepts.

We will now turn our attention to the different type of data and the types of SPC charts associated with each data type. Some readers who are involved in improvement will find this information beyond what they need or want to know. The information is included for those who want to delve more deeply into the topic.

When applying statistical process control methods to healthcare, it is important to recognize and understand the different types of data one encounters. Data are the actual pieces of information that are collected or observed during the process of delivering care. For example, if you ask five physicians how many inpatients they are managing, they might provide you the following data: 0, 3, 1, 5 and 16 (the latter physician might be a hospitalist who covers an intensive care unit). These represent examples of discrete data. Not all data are numbers. For example, if you record the gender of each of the patients in a physician's practice, you might get the following data: male, female, female, male and female.

Most data fall into one of two groups: *categorical* (or attribute) data and *numerical* data. The characteristics of these data types are illustrated in Figure 107.

Categorical data		Numerical data	
Nominal	Ordinal	Discrete	Continuous
Values or observations can be assigned a code in the form of a number where the numbers are simply labels. You can count but not order or measure nominal data. Examples: sex, eye color, etc.	Values or observations can be ranked (put in order) or have a rating scale attached. You can count and order but not measure ordinal data. Examples: low/medium/high, poor/good/excellent, Stage I/Stage II/ Stage III, etc.	Values or observations can be counted (1, 2, 3...) and are distinct and separate. Examples: the number of patients on a panel, the number of doses of a medication delivered, the number of instruments counted, etc.	You can measure continuous data. Values or observations may take on any value within a finite or infinite interval. Examples: height, weight, time, temperature, etc.

Figure 107: Data types

Categorical (attribute) data

Categorical data are observed variables that can be sorted into groups or categories based on their characteristics or attributes. Another name for categorical data is *qualitative* data. There are two types of categorical data seen in healthcare: *nominal data* and *ordinal data*.

As the name implies, nominal data refer to named categories. Nominal data are items that are differentiated by a simple naming system based on their observed characteristics or attributes, such as a person's gender, marital status, ethnicity, birth date or a DRG category.

Nominal data often have two categories ("alive" or "dead," "male" or "female," "present" or "absent"). That is, it is binary. Nominal data can take on numerical values (such as "1" indicating male and "2" indicating female), but those numbers do not have mathematical meaning. For instance, you cannot add 1's and 2's for male and female together and have it make any sense. This type of data are most often summarized with counts, proportions or rates. For example, "a proportional of the total" is binary. Nominal data in binary form generally have a *binomial frequency distribution*. Proportion charts (p charts) are often used to describe attribute data. These represent the most common type of control chart in healthcare. There are also specific statistical tests that are used in analyzing nominal data (i.e., X^2 test, Fisher's exact test, etc.).

Ordinal data mix numerical and categorical data. The data fall into categories, but the numbers assigned to the categories have meaning. They are ordered, named categories. Observations on an ordinal scale are set into some kind of order by their position on the scale. Observations may indicate things such as temporal position, superiority, worsening, etc. For example, rating a hospital or clinic on a scale from 0 stars (lowest) to 5 stars (highest) represents ordinal data. Other examples of ordinal data include low/medium/high, Stage I/Stage II/Stage III/Stage IV, and poor/fair/good/very good/excellent. Ordinal data are often treated as categorical, where the groups are ordered when graphs and charts are made. However, ordinal data contain more information than nominal data. Unlike categorical data, the numbers do have mathematical meaning. For example, if you survey 100 people and ask them to rate a hospital on a scale from 0 to 5, taking the average of the 100 responses will have meaning. This would not be the case with nominal data. This type of data is generally summarized with counts, proportions or rates. An example of a statistical test used in analyzing ordinal data is the Jonckheere-Terpstra test. The Jonckheere-Terpstra test takes advantage of the ordered categories. Therefore, it has more power than the statistical tests used on nominal data (e.g., X^2 test, Fisher's exact test). From a practical perspective, more statistical power means a test can extract more information and is better able to detect assignable variation when it does occur.

Numerical data

These data have meaning as a measurement, such as a person's height, weight, IQ or blood pressure. Alternatively, they are a count, such as the number of patients in a physician panel, an instrument count following surgery or how many patients a physician can see in a clinic every day. Statisticians often refer to numerical data as *quantitative data*. Numerical data can be further broken into two types: *discrete* and *continuous*.

- Discrete data represent items that can be counted. The most common form of discrete data are the cardinal numbering system (0, 1, 2, 3,), which is commonly used in healthcare. Discrete variables are measured across a set of fixed values, such as age in years (not microseconds). A person will say, "I am 20 years old" — not, "I am 20.672 years old." These are often arbitrary scales, such as scoring one's level of satisfaction, although such scales can also be continuous.

- Continuous data represent measurements. These measures are tracked along a continuous scale that can be divided into fractions or described down to multiple decimal points, such as temperature. Continuous variables allow for infinitely fine subdivisions, which means that if your measurements are sufficiently accurate, you can compare two items and determine the difference.

There are two types of numerical data that are most often seen in healthcare: interval data and ratio data.

Interval data are measured along a scale in which each position is equidistant from the one before and after it. This allows for the distance between two pairs to be equivalent. Examples of interval data include a satisfaction scale rated from 1 to 10, temperature in degrees Fahrenheit and dates on a calendar. This type of data contain more information than ordinal data. Interval data are generally described using intervals on a real number line. Interval data do not have a meaningful zero. As a result, interval data cannot be multiplied or divided. The values for interval data cannot be counted, nor can they form meaningful ratios. Interval data are usually summarized using means and variances (standard deviations). An example of interval data is the Celsius or Fahrenheit temperature scale. A person's temperature generally ranges from 95 degrees to 105 degrees Fahrenheit. At any given time, one's temperature can be 98.6 degrees, 99.2 degrees or any one of numerous other points along the temperature scale. Interval data are uncommon and rarely part of an improvement project in healthcare.

Ratio data are numbers that can form meaningful ratios. Examples in healthcare include weight, age, blood pressure, and cost. Ratio data can be either continuous (e.g., can take on any numeric value, such as cost or weight) or discrete (e.g., meaningful only at discrete values, such as number of children). Ratio data contain more information than interval, ordinal or nominal data. In a ratio scale, numbers can be compared as multiples of one another.

For example, a person can be twice as tall as another person. In addition, the number zero has meaning. Thus, the difference between a person of 35 and a person of 38 is the same as the difference between people who are 15 and 18. A person can also have an age of zero. Ratio data can be multiplied or divided because the difference between 1 and 2 is the same as the difference between 3 and 4, and, 4 is twice as much as 2. This type of data are summarized with means and variances (standard deviations). Statistical tests that use ratio data include ANOVA and regression analysis.

Parametric and nonparametric distributions

There are a variety of different SPC charts. The choice of which SPC chart you use depends on the underlying frequency distribution of the data type being analyzed. There are two general types of frequency distributions: *parametric* and *nonparametric*.

A parametric distribution is shown in Figure 108. Parametric frequency distributions have an equation that describes the shape of the frequency distribution. The equation has parameters (variables). Most useful distributions have a single parameter that is the mean, or average. A few distributions have two parameters (mean and variance). Some rare distributions add a third parameter (mean, variance and offset from origin).

The characteristics of parametric and nonparametric distributions are shown in Figure 109.

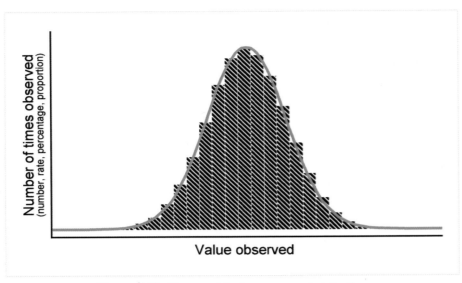

Figure 108: Parametric frequency distribution

Parametric and nonparametric distribution characteristics		
	Parametric	Nonparametric
Assumed distribution	Normal	Any
Assumed variance	Homogenous	Any
Typical data type	Ratio or interval	Nominal or ordinal
Data set relations	Independent	Any
Usual central measure	Mean	Median
Benefits	Can draw more conclusions	Simplicity: less affected by outliers

Figure 109: Parametric and nonparametric distribution characteristics

Statistical resolution or power refers to how well a statistical test can detect differences. Power is determined by data type (i.e., ratio data exceeds interval data, which exceeds ordinal data, which exceeds nominal data). Parametric distributions give better power and resolution than nonparametric distributions, but they make assumptions about the underlying frequency distribution that may or may not be true. This is why you have to understand the data type you are observing and be sure you know what the most likely distribution is for that data. Whenever feasible, you will want to select the highest statistical power possible when analyzing data.

Choosing the appropriate SPC chart

Once different data types are understood, you can look at the different types of statistical process control charts applicable to each data type, as shown in Figure 110. Because interval data are not commonly seen in healthcare improvement projects, the control charts used for this type of data will not be discussed.

The p chart

The p chart ("proportion" chart) is the most common type of control chart in healthcare. It is typically used to look at variation within binary attributes data where there are two possible outcomes (e.g., a defect is present or it is not, a condition is present or it is not). It is used in situations where the sample size is relatively small.

Types of SPC charts commonly used in healthcare			
Data type	Measurement example	Frequency distribution	SPC chart
Attribution (nominal or ordinal) – in binary form (a common situation in healthcare improvement projects)	Acute Myocardial Infarction (AMI) mortality: • Numerator: AMI patients discharged with the state of "expire" • Denominator: all AMI patient discharges	Binomial distribution	Use the p chart — "proportion chart" for small sample sizes where np ≥ 5 Where n = sample size and p = mean proportion
Discrete ratio data – "number of per unit" data	Number of primary bloodstream infections (PBIs) per 1,000 central line days: • Numerator: number of PBIs • Denominator: total number of days a central line is in place for all patients having central lines	Poisson distribution	Use the c chart — "count per unit chart," or a u chart — "counts per proportion chart"
Discrete ratio data – data in the form of "number of between" events	Mortality from community acquired pneumonia (CAP): • Numerator: CAP patients discharged with the state of "expire" • Denominator: number of non-deaths from CAP between each CAP death	Geometric distribution	Use the g chart
Continuous ratio data	Mean: (average) time to initial antibiotic administration: • Numerator: sum of each patient's number of minutes between time of physician's order to initial antibiotic administration time • Denominator: total number of patients receiving initial antibiotic dose	Gaussian (normal) distribution	Use the X-bar and s chart for "mean and standard deviation chart" with sample size parameter set to "1"

Figure 110: Types of SPC charts
(View Appendix C for larger version)

Because the sub-group size can vary, a p chart often shows a proportion of nonconforming observations rather than the actual count. P charts show how the process changes over time. The process attribute (or characteristic) is always described in a binary manner — male/female, yes/no, pass/fail, alive/dead, etc. Because it is possible to set almost anything up as a proportion, you can often analyze data in this binary form. Examples include the proportion of patients in a specific DRG category, entering a specific hospital, of a particular ethnicity, with a particular infection, developing skin ulcers, or with essentially any complication (other than very rare complications, in which case the g chart is used — see the discussion below). In each case, the proportion represents a "yes/no" situation (either this condition exists or it does not) and is therefore binary.

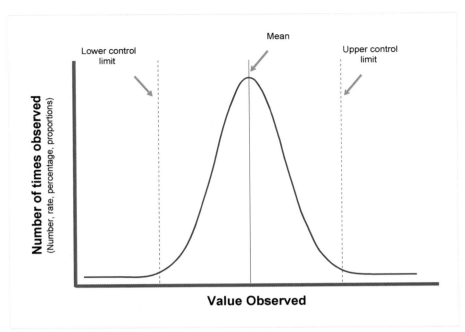

Figure 111: Binominal frequency distribution
(View Appendix C for larger version)

This type of data generates a binomial frequency distribution, as displayed in Figure 111. A binomial distribution looks like a bell-shaped curve (e.g., like a normal distribution). It can get misleading if the distribution is distorted or "skewed" as it nears its binary limits, 0 or 1. This is more likely to happen when the mean proportion and sample size are small. In this circumstance, a Poisson distribution (c chart) may be more appropriate (see discussion of Poisson distributions and c charts below).

There are four properties that indicate a binomial distribution:

1. There are "n" repeated trials or samplings (e.g., a fixed number of observations).

2. All trials are identical and independent.

3. The probability of success is the same for each observation.

4. Each trial has exactly two possible outcomes, "success" and "failure" — that is, it is binary.

The larger the sample size, the more a binomial distribution will approach a true normal distribution. This type of distribution will generate an SPC chart called an X-bar chart (see discussion of Gaussian distributions below).

The g chart

Most of the other types of SPC charts are uncommonly used in healthcare. The g chart is an exception.

Rare events inherently occur in all kinds of processes. In hospitals, there are adverse drug events, unusual post-operative infections, patient falls, ventilator-associated pneumonias, mortality from community-acquired pneumonia, and other rare, adverse events that cause prolonged hospital stays, result in poor outcomes and increase healthcare costs.

Because rare events occur at very low rates, traditional control charts like the p chart are typically not as effective at detecting changes in the event rates in a timely manner. In these situations, the probability that a given event will occur is so low, considerably larger sample sizes are required to create a p chart and abide by the typical rules governing this type of statistical analysis. In addition to the difficult task of collecting more data, this requires the improvement team to wait far longer to detect a significant shift in the process.

The trouble is that when you are considering very rare events, the statistical power depends more on the actual event rate than on your total sample size ("n"). The effective power depends on the number of events.

The g chart is a statistical process control chart developed by James Benneyan to monitor the number of events between rarely occurring errors or nonconforming incidents in healthcare. The g chart creates a picture of a process over time. Each point represents the number of observed units between occurrences of a relatively rare event. For example, deep mediastinal infections following open heart surgery are very rare (incidence of less than 1 percent). If an improvement team focuses on tracking the number

of mediastinal infections, it will take them many years of experience to collect enough cases to have a statistically valid sample. This is also true of other rare events, such as contaminated needle sticks, instances of ventilator associated pneumonia, etc.

To develop a g chart, the team can count and plot the number of non-infection cases occurring between infection cases. This effectively increases the sample size and creates a statistically valid way of analyzing the process. This type of data are summarized with a mean. The "g" in g chart

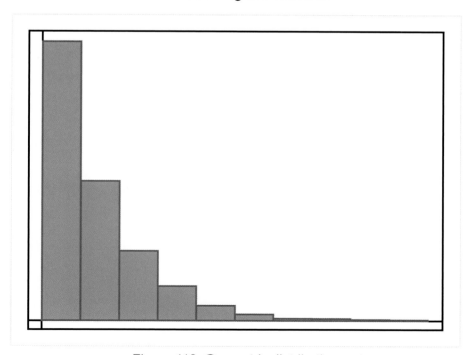

Figure 112: Geometric distribution

stands for geometric, since data relating to events between occurrences is represented by a geometric distribution, as portrayed in Figure 112.

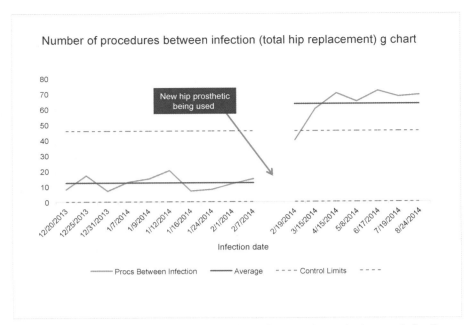

Figure 113: g chart example — number of procedures between infections
(View Appendix C for larger version)

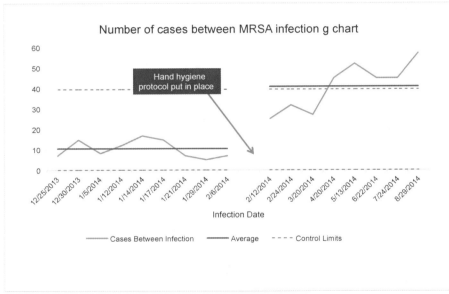

Figure 114: g chart example — MRSA infection
(View Appendix C for larger version)

The g chart helps to display this data in traditional control chart form. Specific formulas for g chart control limits are used with this type of data.

Figure 113 is an example of a g chart illustrating the time between infections in patients receiving total hip replacement. Note the improvement in performance resulting from a change in process (new type of hip prosthesis used).

Figure 114 is an example of a g chart illustrating the time between MRSA infections on a hospital ward as a result of implementing a hand hygiene protocol.

The c chart

It is not uncommon in healthcare to encounter discrete ratio data in the form of "number of per." Examples include number of children per family, number of tests per patient, number of patients per hour, number of patients through a unit per day, number of blood stream infections per 1,000 central line days and so forth. Data of this type follows a Poisson distribution, as illustrated in Figure 115. When you encounter "number of counts per" data, it always suggests a Poisson distribution.

A Poisson frequency distribution has only one parameter, the mean. With a Poisson distribution, the mean equals the standard deviation.

The control chart that corresponds to a Poisson distribution is the c chart (a "count per unit" chart). If the data are expressed as a proportion, the output is called a u chart (a "unit per proportion" chart). Like other control charts, flipping a Poisson distribution on its side and plotting observations over time will generate a c chart or u chart.

The X-bar chart

Continuous ratio data are the fourth type of data commonly encountered in healthcare. Continuous ratio data are summarized by the mean and standard deviation. This type of data almost always yields a normal (Gaussian or bell-shaped) distribution. If it is a near perfect normal distribution, the chart that works with it is called an X-bar chart.

This type of distribution has more than one parameter. X-bar charts generally have two parallel charts, one for the mean and one for the standard deviation (the two parameters that summarize continuous ratio data). In this format, these are called X-bar and s charts. With an X-bar chart, you typically plot every observation.

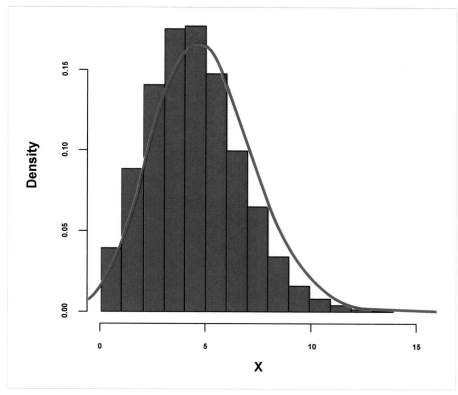

Figure 115: Poisson frequency distribution

What if nothing fits?

There are instances when the data observed in a situation does not easily fit one of the above scenarios. In such situations, the improvement team faces four possible solutions.

① Transform the data. Many healthcare variables do not meet the assumptions of parametric statistical tests. That is, they are not normally distributed, the variances are not homogenous, or both. These frequency distributions frequently are "skewed" — that is, they have a tail, as portrayed in Figure 116. In this type of skewed

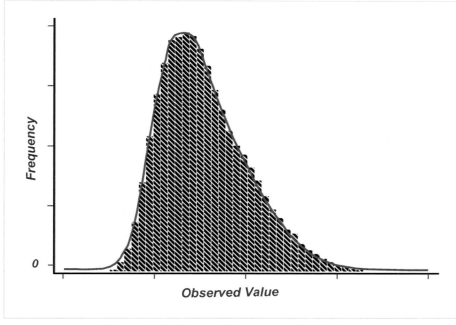

Figure 116: Skewed frequency distribution

distribution, a normal distribution simply does not fit. To "transform" the data, you can perform a mathematical operation on each observation and then use the transformed numbers in a statistical test. If you are going to use one of these transform methods, you need to have a fairly high degree of certainty that your collected data represents a true, clean process (i.e., not a combination of different processes mixed together).

In these situations, there are several types of mathematical transformations you can perform on the data, including:

> Log transforms. This is the most common method for transforming data. You plot the logarithm of each of the data points in the data set. This creates a new frequency distribution that is often a bell-shaped curve, or at least it is less skewed than the initial frequency distribution. When this happens, you can apply parametric tools (e.g., X bar S chart). As a result, patterns in the data become more identifiable and interpretable. Even though you have performed a statistical test on the transformed data, it is not a good idea to report the means, standard errors, or similar results of transformed units. Instead, you need to "back transform" the results by doing the opposite of the mathematical function that was initially used in the data transformation. In a log transformation, a back transform is done by raising 10 to the power of the calculated mean of the logarithmic distribution. The upper and lower control limits, and the individual data points, can be similarly back transformed. While it is good to understand this technique conceptually, it is not necessary to understand the mathematics involved. Suffice it to say that the process has been shown to be mathematically legitimate. Taking this approach does not result in any loss of statistical power.

> Power transforms. If a log transform does not work, a "root" or "power" transform can be done. This is generally the third square root of your X's, the fifth square root of your X's, or the seventh square root of your X's. Once again, this process can often transform skewed results into a more normal distribution, allowing you to apply parametric tools. Once these tools have been applied, you need to back transform the data, mean and control limits in a fashion similar to that mentioned under log transforms above. Taking this approach does not result in any loss of statistical power.

> Use severity of illness transforms. Technically, severity of illness adjustments can be viewed as a type of transformation. Severity of illness adjustments attempt to eliminate variation arising from differences among patients by breaking a cohort of patients into a series of sub-groups that are relatively homogenous in terms of severity based on a particular measurement parameter (e.g., cost

per case or risk of mortality). If you break a skewed distribution of patients into severity of illness categories in this fashion, it is not uncommon to find that the skewed distribution is actually composed of a series of normal distributions — a normal distribution for each category of severity in the cohort of patients under observation, as seen in Figure

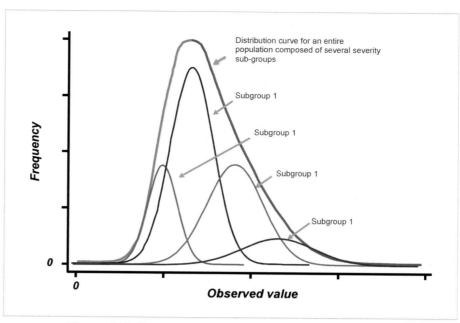

Figure 117: Parametric distributions based on severity
(View Appendix C for larger version)

117. You can then do the analysis on each subset of parametric distributions. Once this is done, they can be mathematically rolled back together. You do not lose any statistical power with this approach.

> Linear, cyclic, or nonlinear transforms. There are a variety of other mathematical transformations that can be performed on unusual frequency distributions to enable the application of parametric techniques. A detailed discussion of these methods is beyond the scope of this discussion.

❷ Use Shewhart's method of addressing a non-homogenous sample. Whenever possible, Shewhart sought to convert a data sample into a dataset that would generate a normal distribution to which parametric methods could be applied. In a non-homogenous population, as illustrated in Figure 118, you can randomly draw patients in small groups out of

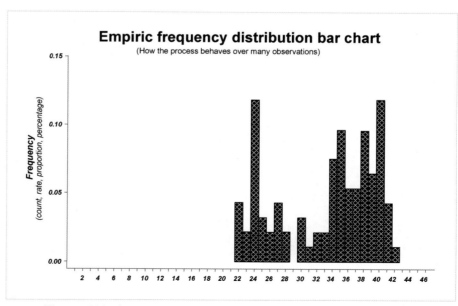

Figure 118: Shewhart's method for non-homogenous samples
(View Appendix C for larger version)

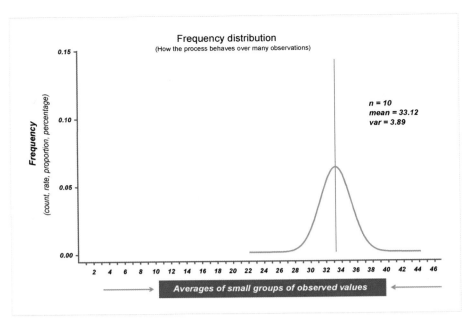

Figure 119: Shewhart's method for non-homogenous frequency distribution (View Appendix C for larger version)

the total non-homogenous population and create frequency distributions for each of these random groups. If you do this a large number of times (or more accurately, get a computer to do it a large number of times), you can plot averages of small groups of observed values. This generally results in a normal distribution to which you can apply parametric techniques, as shown in Figure 119. Using this approach maintains statistical power. This is an example of the so-called central limit theorem.

❸ Use some other known frequency distribution. There are many of these, but most are very esoteric and not pertinent to healthcare except for highly unusual situations.

❹ Use a non-parametric control chart—an XmR control chart. The problem with this approach is that you will lose a lot of statistical power. XmR charts provide the lowest level of statistical power. As a result, this is a choice of last resort.

For those involved in clinical and operational improvement, it is not necessary to understand the complicated mathematics behind these methods. You can always get a statistician or a computer to do the computations. However, it is important to understand the rules and techniques at a conceptual level in order to make the appropriate directional decisions when you encounter datasets that require the application of these methods.

There are a number of sources that provide a more detailed discussion of the different types of frequency distributions and their associated SPC charts, as well as their respective uses in healthcare. The interested reader can consult these other sources for additional information.[157, 158, 159]

APPENDIX C: FIGURES

Chapter 4

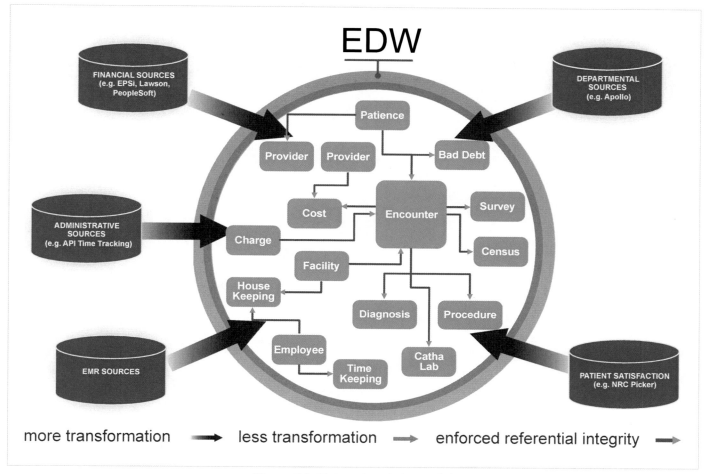

Figure 26: Enterprise data model

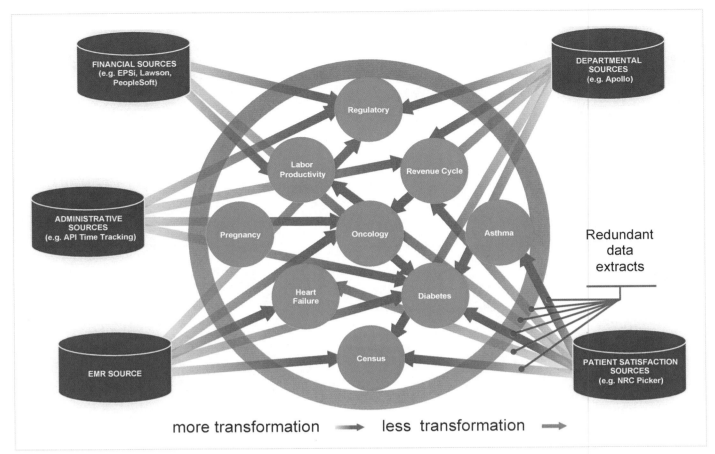

Figure 27: Dimensional data model

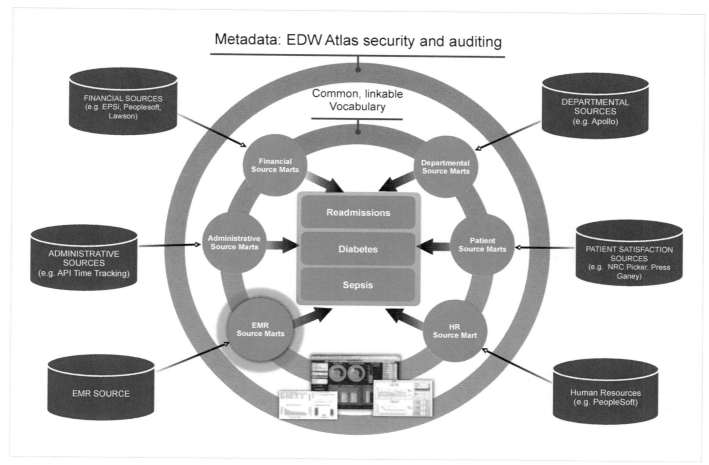

Figure 28: Late-Binding™ Data Warehouse

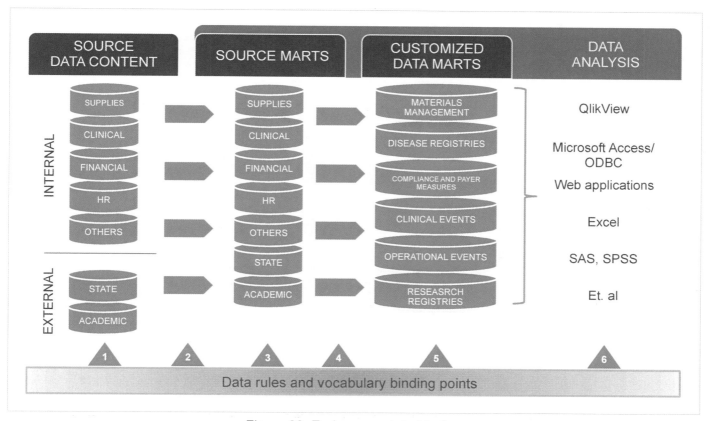

Figure 29: Early versus late binding

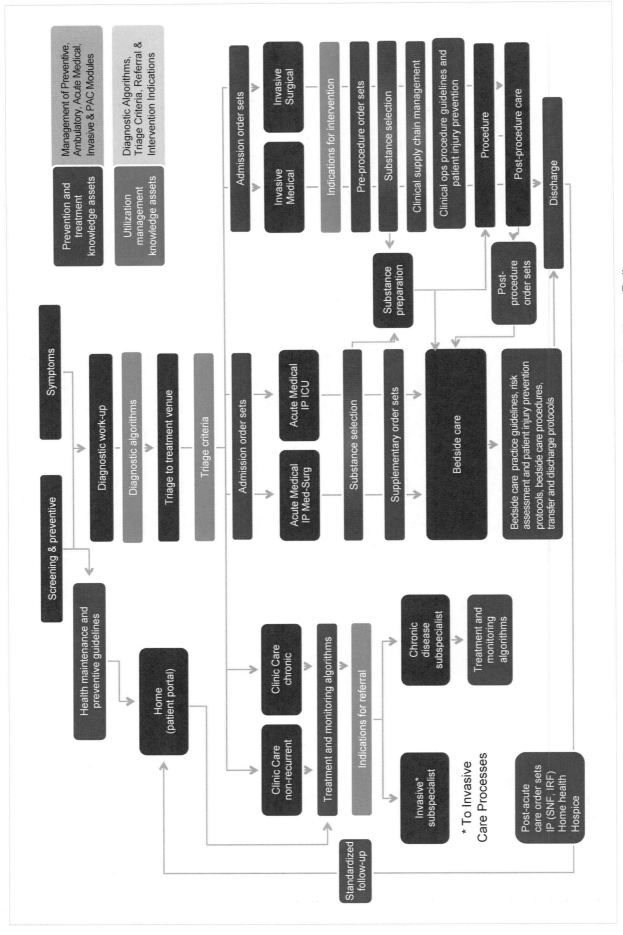

Figure 32: Population health management — Anatomy of Healthcare Delivery

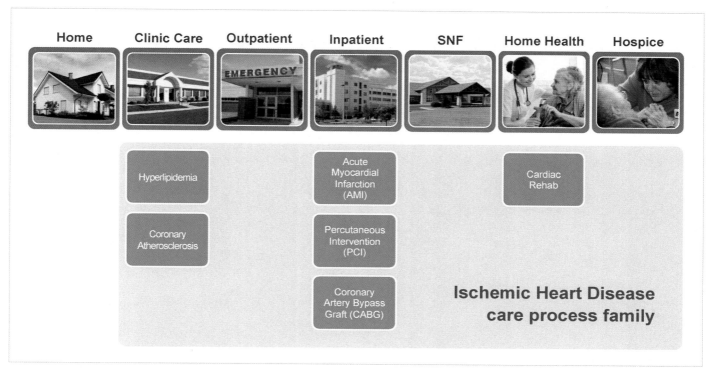

Figure 33: Clinical Integration hierarchy — care process families

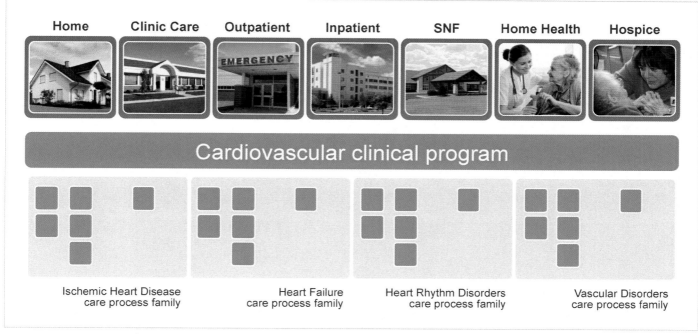

Figure 34: Clinical Integration hierarchy — cardiovascular clinical program

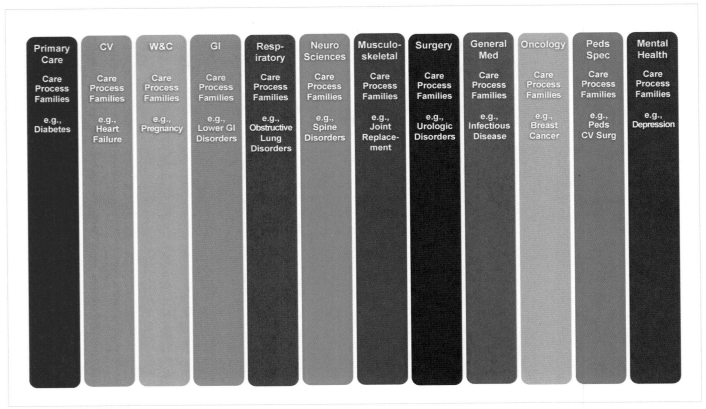

Figure 35: Clinical programs — ordering of care

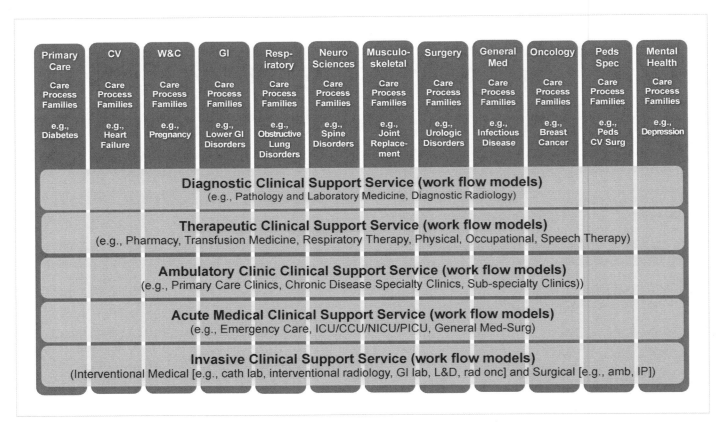

Figure 36: Clinical support services — delivery of care

Value Stream Map	Diagnostic CSS			Ambulatory CSS		Acute Medical CSS			Invasive CSS		
	Clin Path	Anat Path	Radi-ology	Peds	Adult	ECU	ICU/CCU	Med-Surg	IP Surg	ASC	Interv Med
Substances											
Pharmacy				X	X	X	X	X	X	X	X
Medications			X	X	X	X	X	X	X	X	X
Fluids						X	X	X	X	X	X
Electrolytes				X	X	X	X	X	X	X	X
Parenteral nutrition (TPN)						X	X	X	X		
Transfusion Medicine						X	X	X	X		
Glycemic Control (Glucose Mgmt)							X	X	X	X	
Healthcare Associated Infections											
Ventilator Associated Pneumonia							X				
Urinary Catheter Infections						X	X	X	X	X	X
Surgical Site Infections									X	X	X
Central Line Assoc Bldstream Inf						X	X	X	X		
Venous Thromboembolism							X	X	X	X	
Pressure Injury (Decubitus Ulcers)							X	X			
Falls (Strength, Agility, Cognition)						X	X	X			
Patient/Procedure Control									X	X	

Figure 37: Value stream protocols to help prevent patient injuries

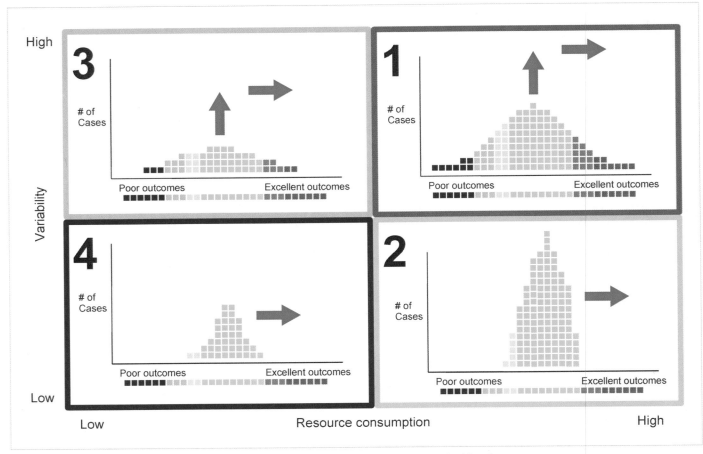

Figure 50: Improvement approach — prioritization

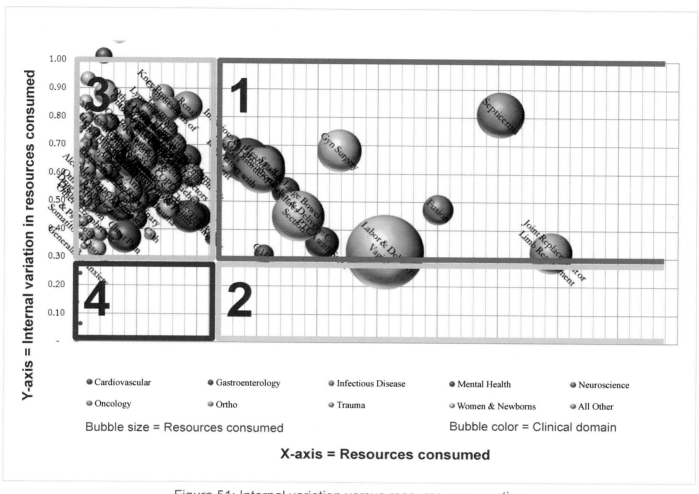

Figure 51: Internal variation versus resource consumption

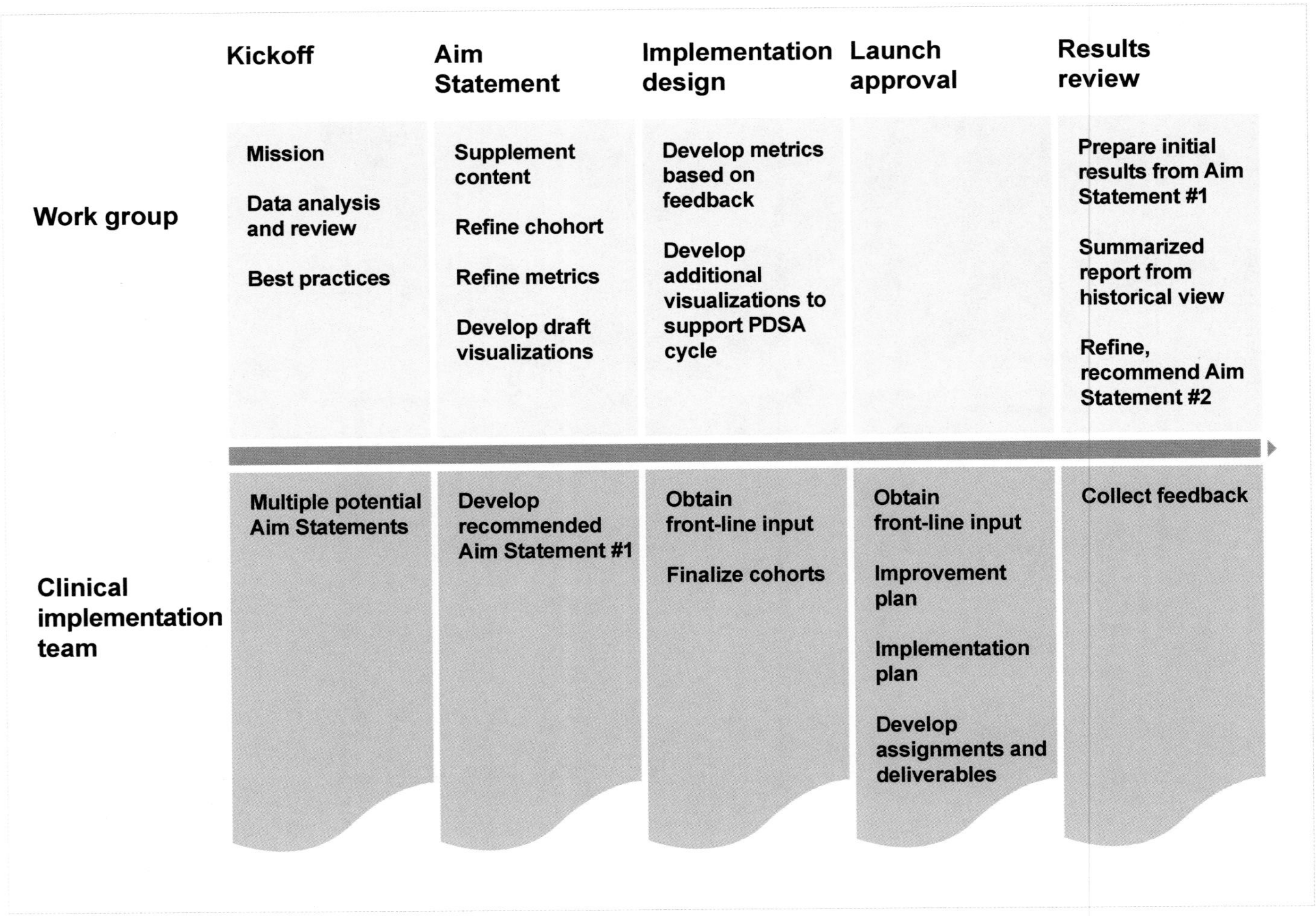

	Kickoff	Aim Statement	Implementation design	Launch approval	Results review
Work group	Mission Data analysis and review Best practices	Supplement content Refine chohort Refine metrics Develop draft visualizations	Develop metrics based on feedback Develop additional visualizations to support PDSA cycle		Prepare initial results from Aim Statement #1 Summarized report from historical view Refine, recommend Aim Statement #2
Clinical implementation team	Multiple potential Aim Statements	Develop recommended Aim Statement #1	Obtain front-line input Finalize cohorts	Obtain front-line input Improvement plan Implementation plan Develop assignments and deliverables	Collect feedback

Figure 58: Standard organizational workflow

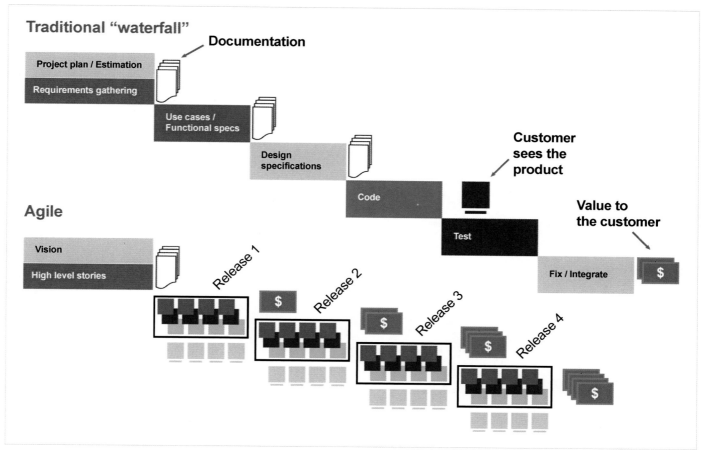

Figure 60: Traditional versus Agile development approach

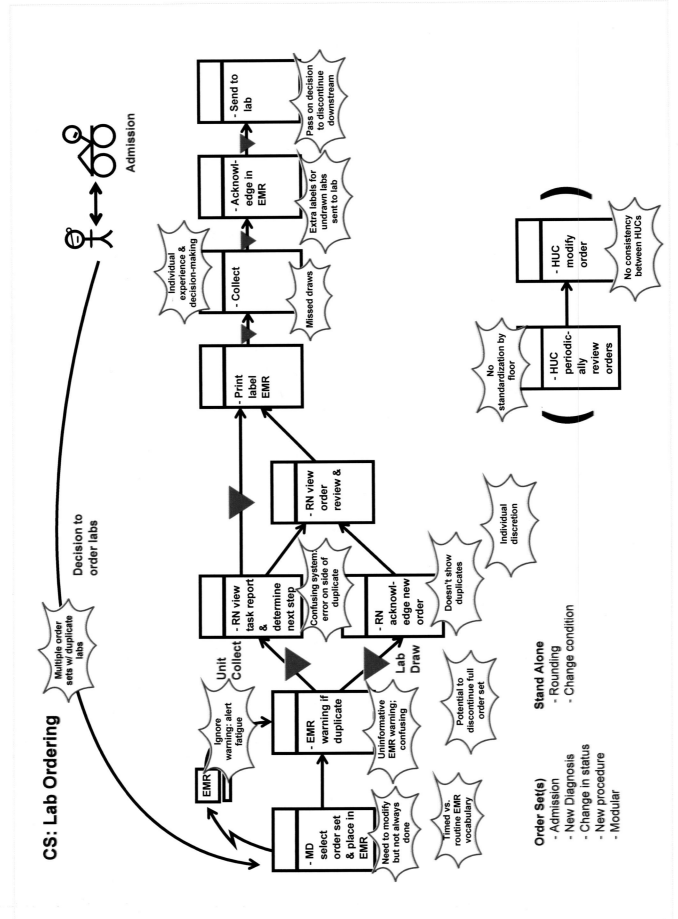

Figure 62: Using Lean to identify challenges

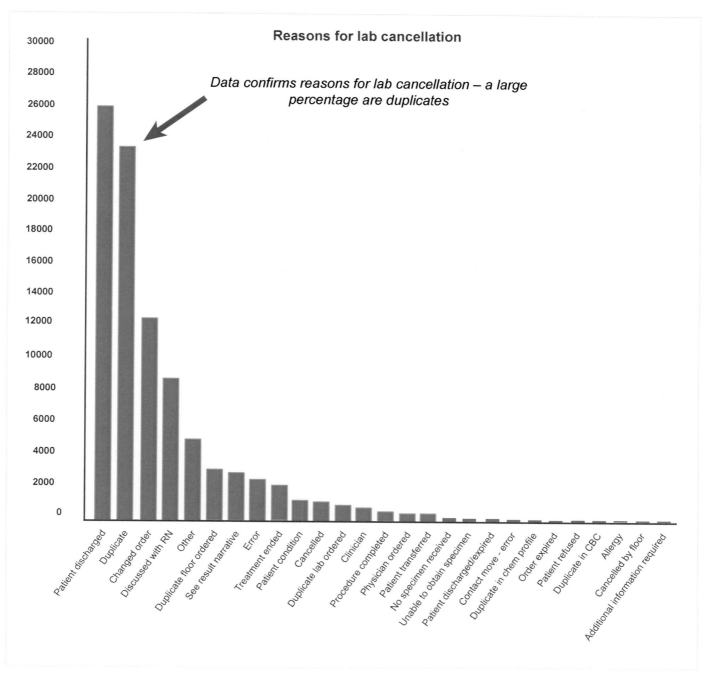

Figure 64: Lab cancellation example

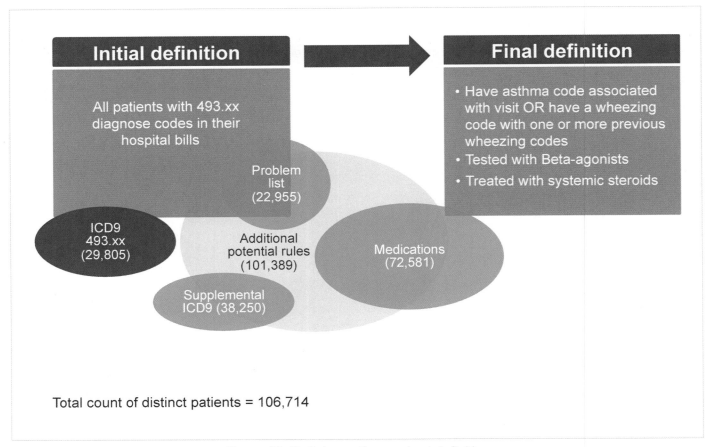

Figure 66: Defining asthma cohort definition

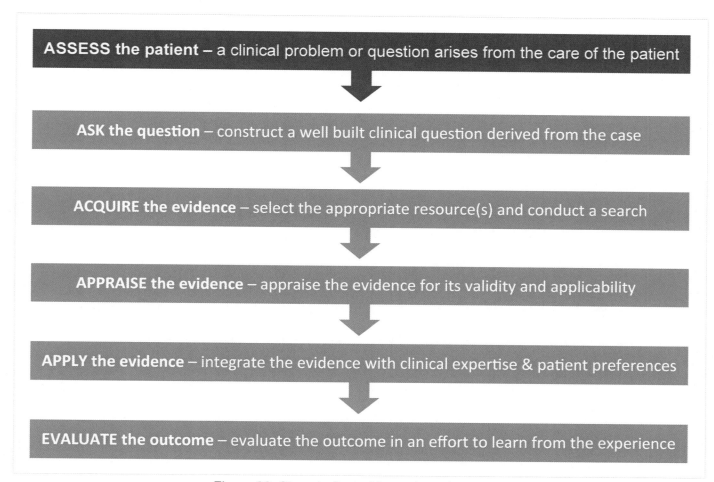

Figure 68: Steps in the evidence-based process

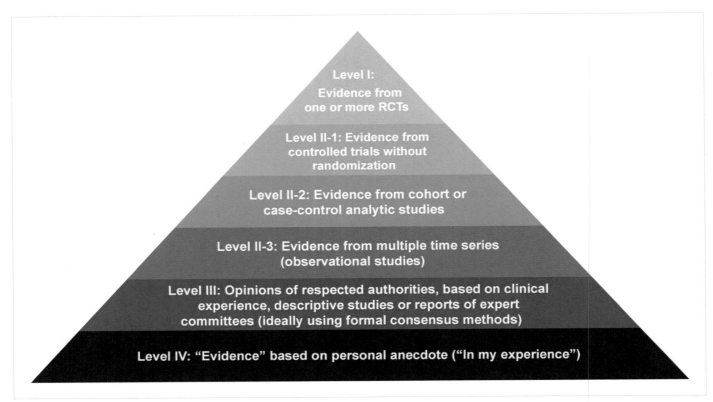

Figure 69: Levels of evidence

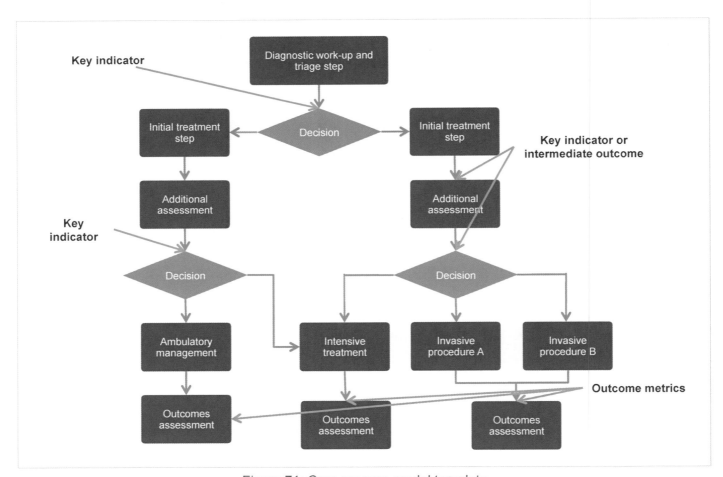

Figure 71: Care process model template

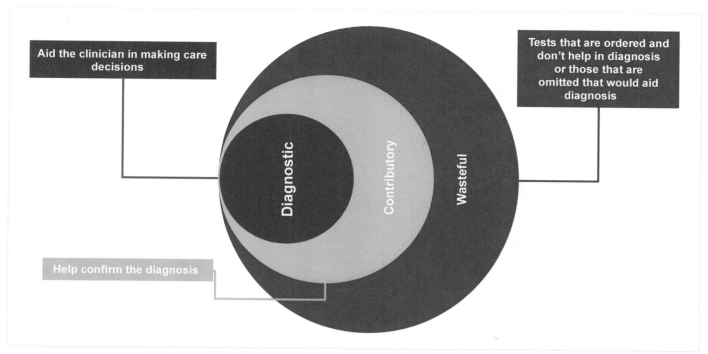

Figure 74: Ordering waste — diagnostic tests

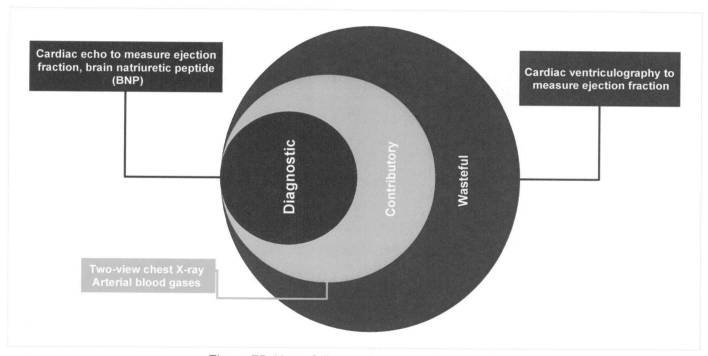

Figure 75: Heart failure ordering waste example

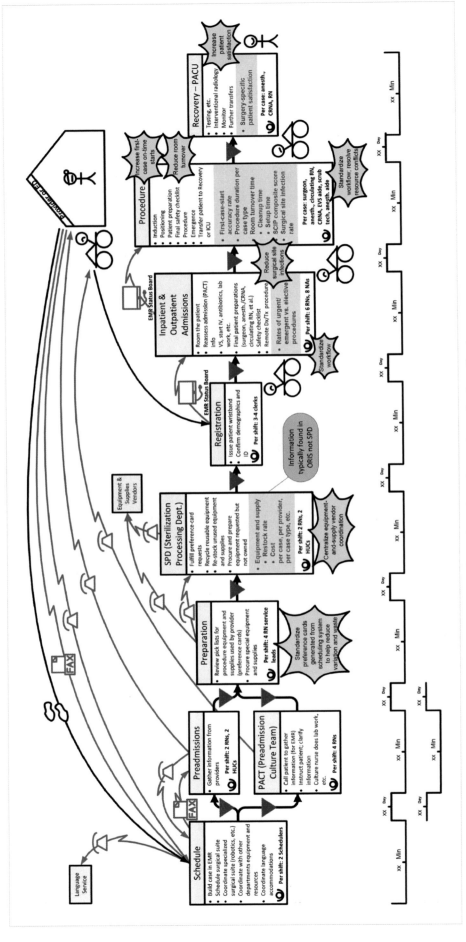

Figure 77: Sample value stream map for inpatient surgery

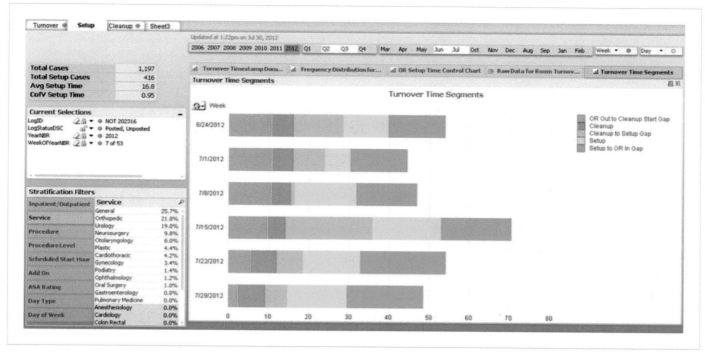

Figure 78: Operating room workflow

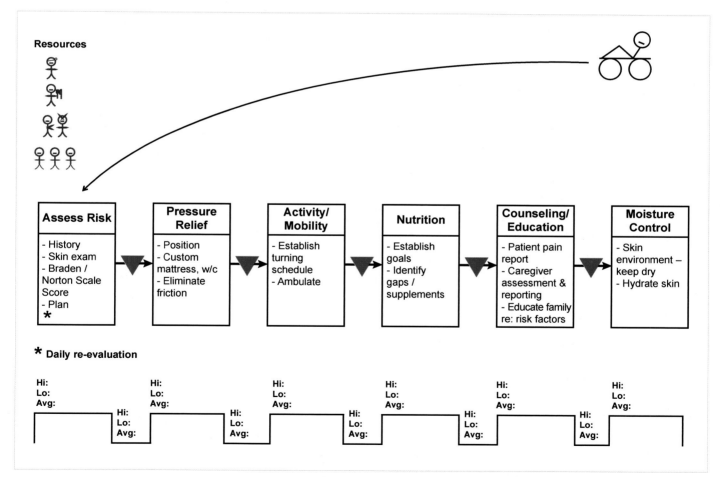

Figure 79: Pressure injury prevention

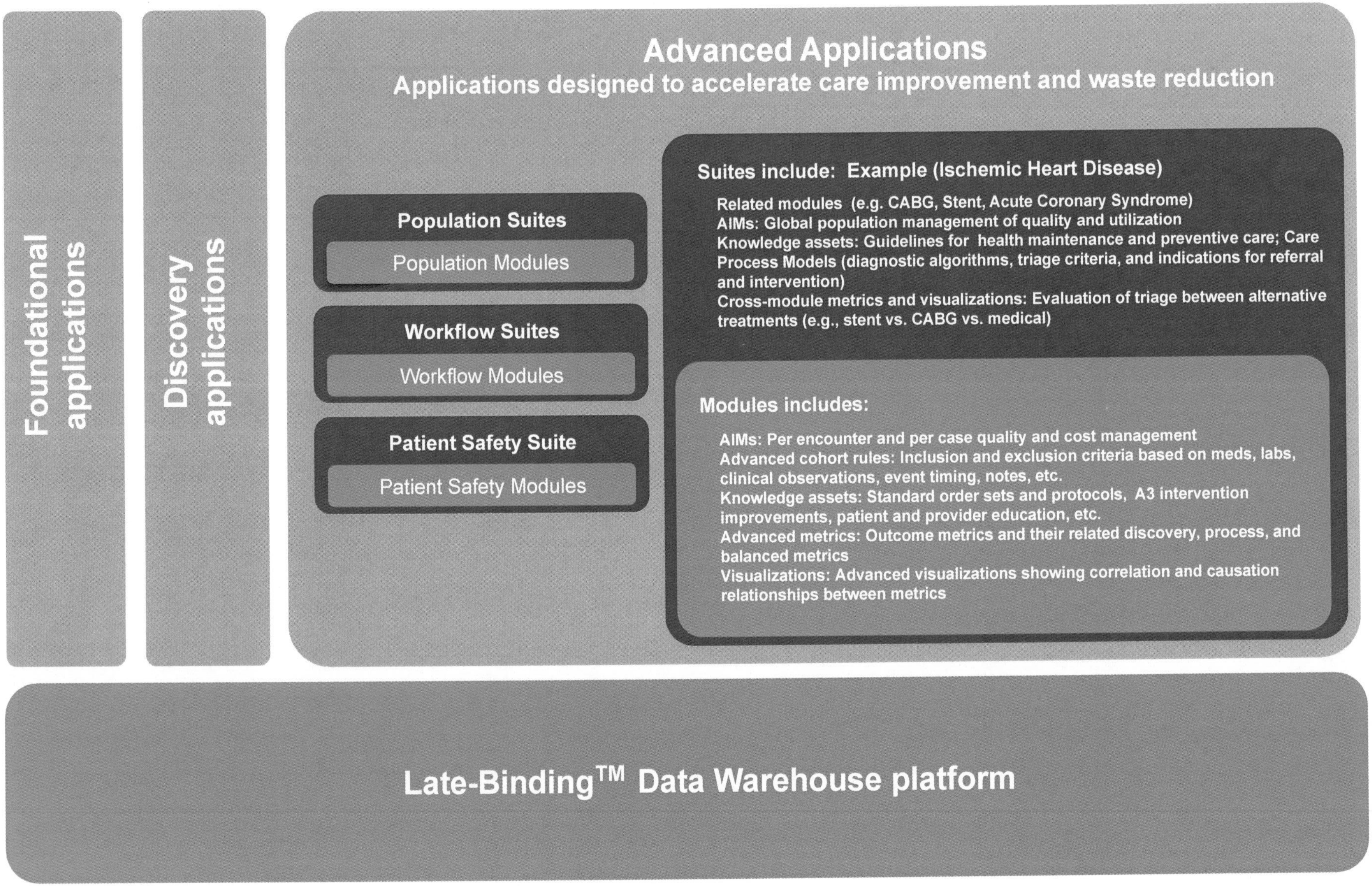

Advanced Applications

Applications designed to accelerate care improvement and waste reduction

Suites include: Example (Ischemic Heart Disease)

Related modules (e.g. CABG, Stent, Acute Coronary Syndrome)
AIMs: Global population management of quality and utilization
Knowledge assets: Guidelines for health maintenance and preventive care; Care
Process Models (diagnostic algorithms, triage criteria, and indications for referral
and intervention)
Cross-module metrics and visualizations: Evaluation of triage between alternative
treatments (e.g., stent vs. CABG vs. medical)

Modules includes:

AIMs: Per encounter and per case quality and cost management
Advanced cohort rules: Inclusion and exclusion criteria based on meds, labs,
clinical observations, event timing, notes, etc.
Knowledge assets: Standard order sets and protocols, A3 intervention
improvements, patient and provider education, etc.
Advanced metrics: Outcome metrics and their related discovery, process, and
balanced metrics
Visualizations: Advanced visualizations showing correlation and causation
relationships between metrics

Population Suites

Population Modules

Workflow Suites

Workflow Modules

Patient Safety Suite

Patient Safety Modules

Discovery applications

Foundational applications

Late-Binding™ Data Warehouse platform

Figure 84: Health Catalyst Advanced Applications

Types of flow charts:

- **Work-flow** – physical flow of people, work, documents, information
- **Deployment** – flow of work processes and individual responsibilities (matrix diagram)
- **Outline** – describes principal features of a process
- **Top-down,** hierarchical – helps show systems
- **Detailed** – most time consuming (industrial model)

Examples of symbols used

Symbol	Description	Symbol	Description
	Terminal (Marks the beginning and ending of a process)		Delay symbol (indicates wait time until next step occurs)
	Activity/process (Single step in the process)	on-page on-page	Connectors (flowchart continues elsewhere)
	Decision (Decision must be made - yes or no)	→	Flow lines (sequential steps in the process)

Figure 85: Types of flow charts and flow chart symbols

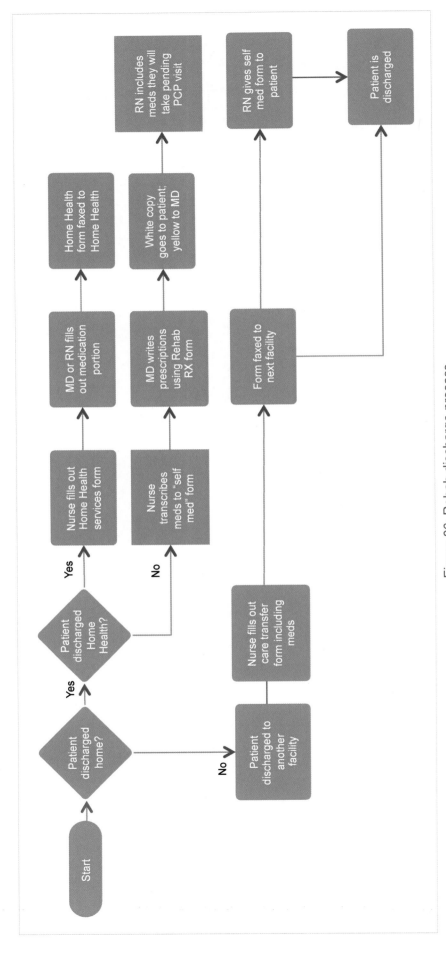

Figure 86: Rehab discharge process

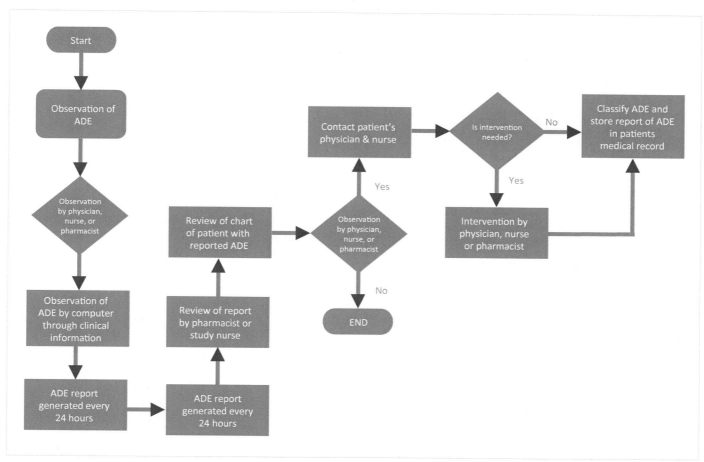

Figure 87: Detection of adverse drug events process

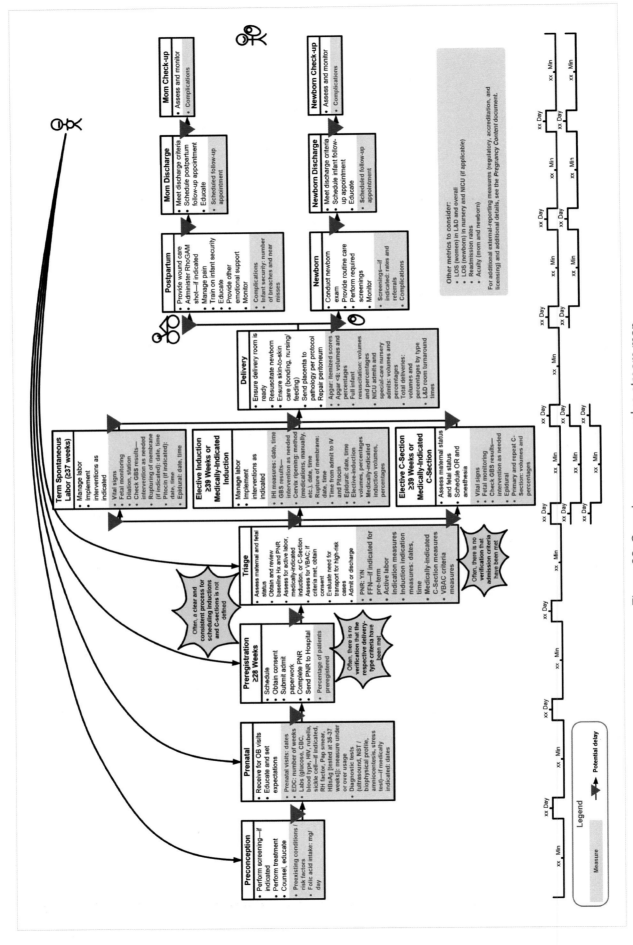

Figure 88: Sample pregnancy value stream map

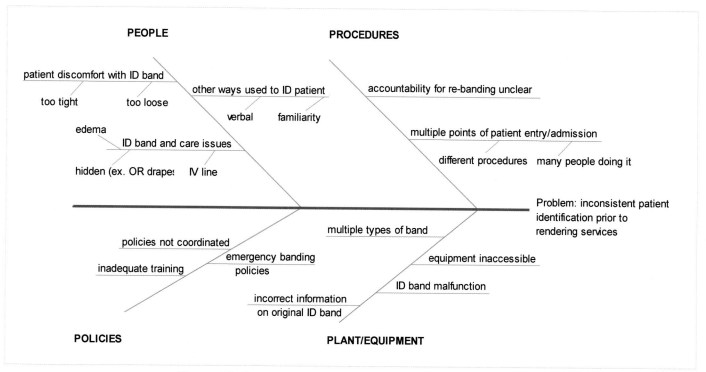

Figure 89: Sample patient identification fishbone diagram

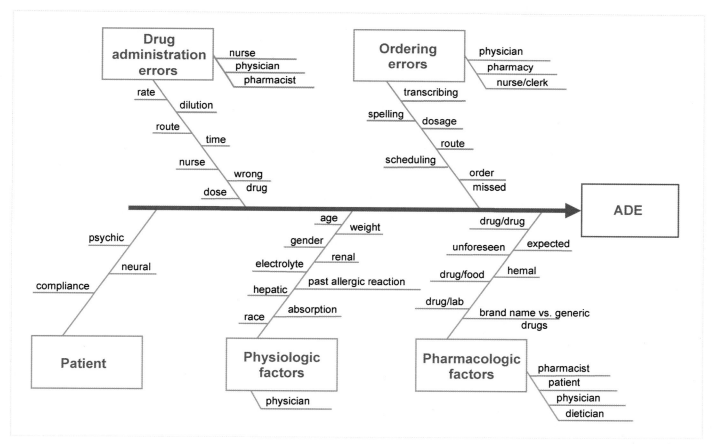

Figure 90: Sample adverse drug effects fishbone diagram

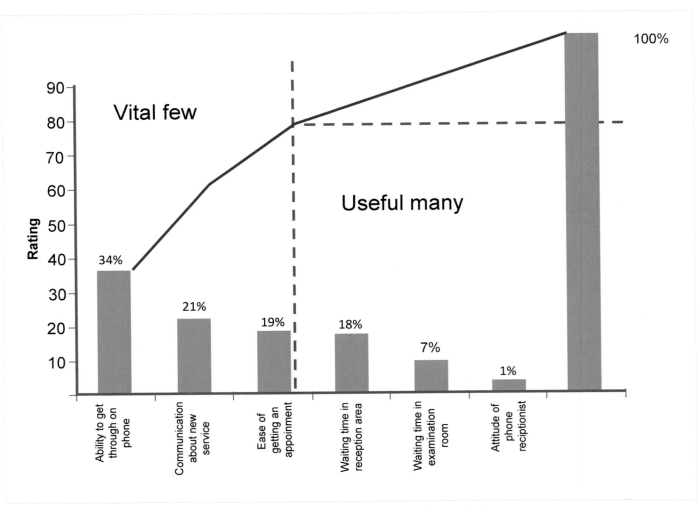

Figure 92: Pareto analysis — family practice patient survey

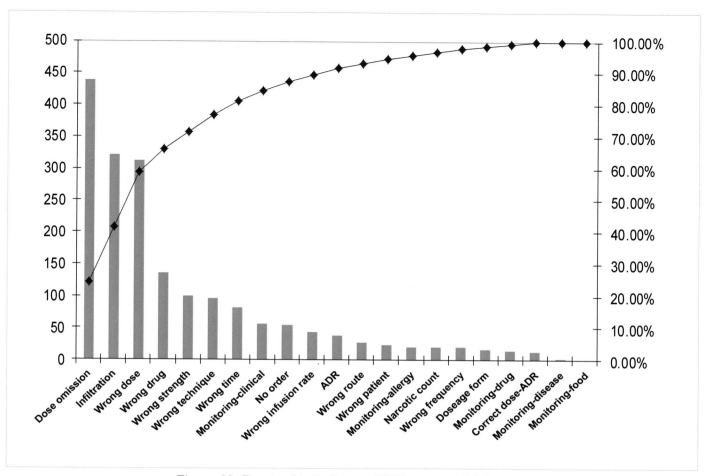

Figure 93: Pareto distribution — 2007 reported ADE types

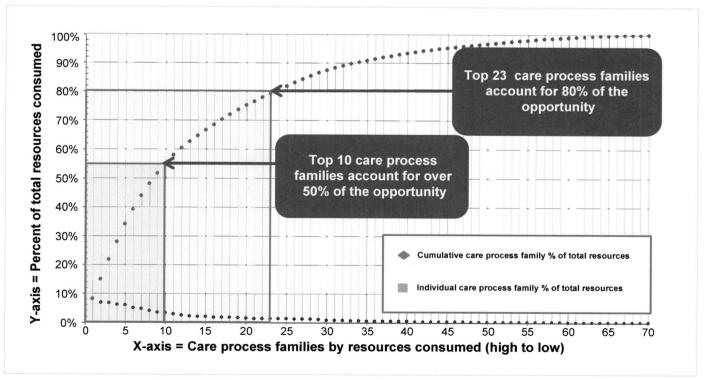

Figure 94: Key Process Analysis

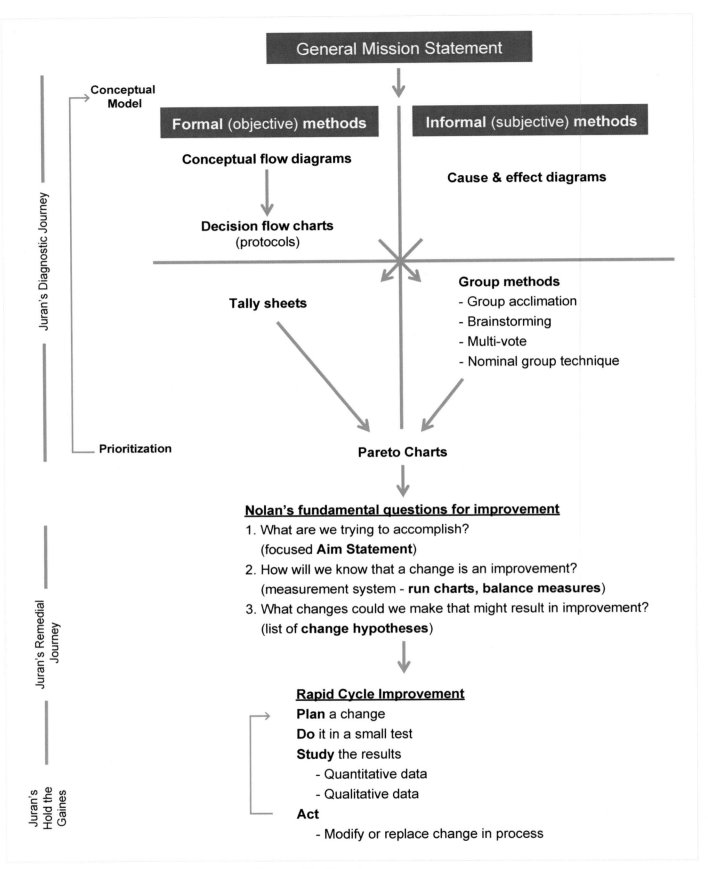

Figure 97: Modeling processes

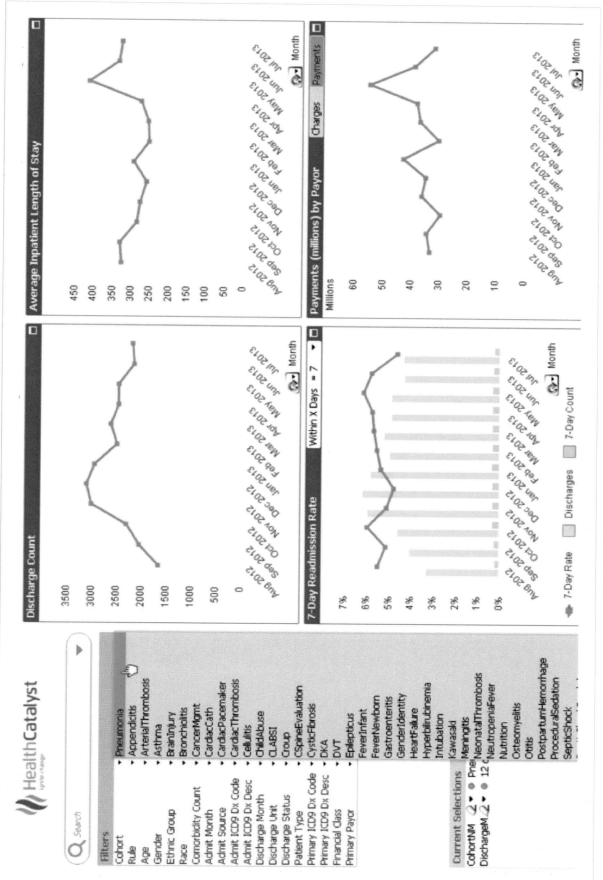

Chapter 7

Figure 98: Sample Population Explorer visualization

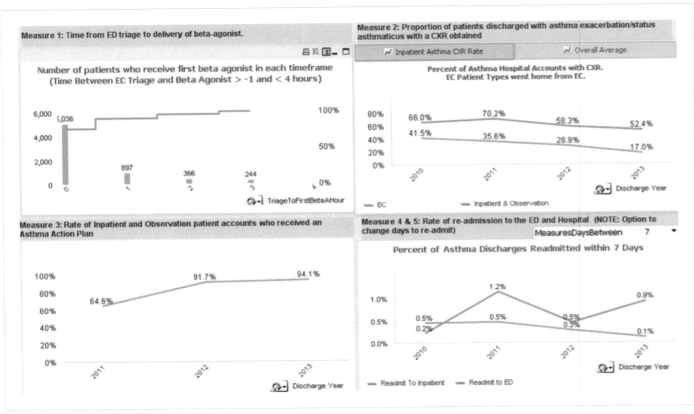

Figure 99: Sample asthma visualization

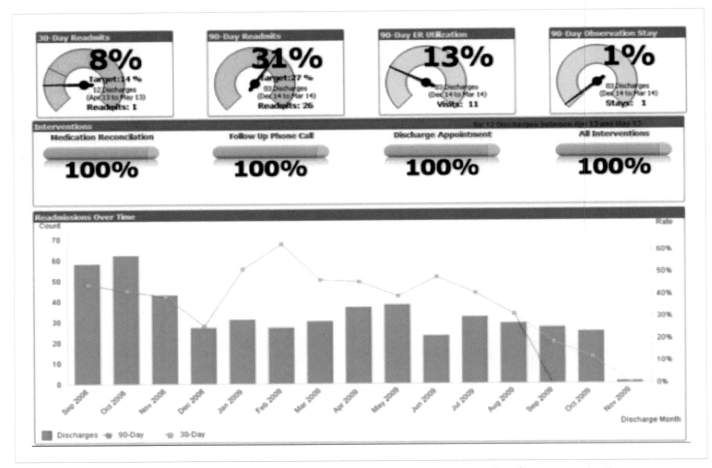

Figure 100: Sample heart failure readmission visualization

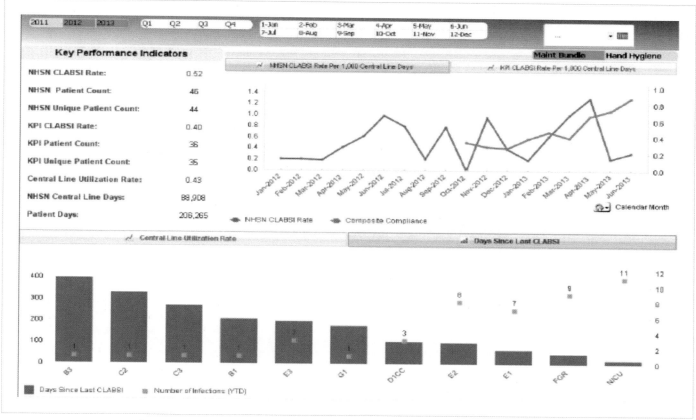

Figure 101: Sample CLABSI visualization

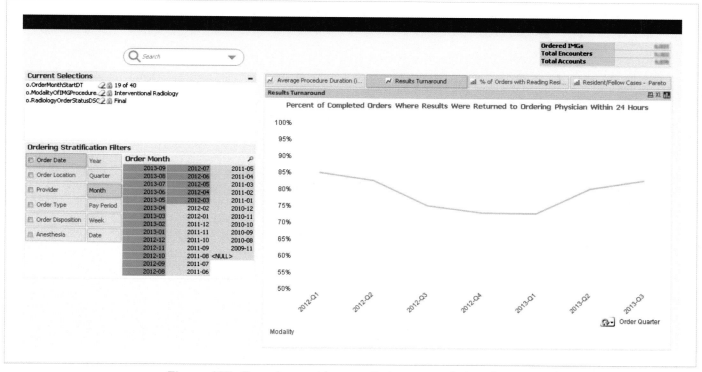

Figure 102: Sample provider results turnaround visualization

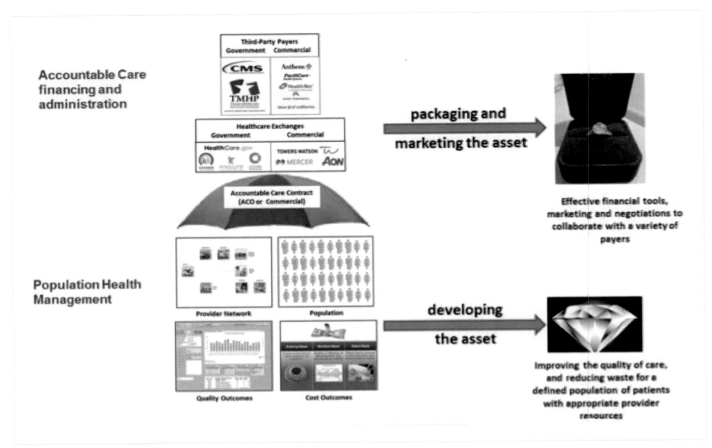

Chapter 8

Figure 103: ACO model

Types of SPC charts commonly used in healthcare			
Data type	Measurement example	Frequency distribution	SPC chart
Attribution (nominal or ordinal) – in binary form (a common situation in healthcare improvement projects)	Acute Myocardial Infarction (AMI) mortality: • Numerator: AMI patients discharged with the state of "expire" • Denominator: all AMI patient discharges	Binomial distribution	Use the p chart — "proportion chart" for small sample sizes where $np \geq 5$ Where n = sample size and p = mean proportion
Discrete ratio data – "number of per unit" data	Number of primary bloodstream infections (PBIs) per 1,000 central line days: • Numerator: number of PBIs • Denominator: total number of days a central line is in place for all patients having central lines	Poisson distribution	Use the c chart — "count per unit chart," or a u chart — "counts per proportion chart"
Discrete ratio data – data in the form of "number of between" events	Mortality from community acquired pneumonia (CAP): • Numerator: CAP patients discharged with the state of "expire" • Denominator: number of non-deaths from CAP between each CAP death	Geometric distribution	Use the g chart
Continuous ratio data	Mean: (average) time to initial antibiotic administration: • Numerator: sum of each patient's number of minutes between time of physician's order to initial antibiotic administration time • Denominator: total number of patients receiving initial antibiotic dose	Gaussian (normal) distribution	Use the X-bar and s chart for "mean and standard deviation chart" with sample size parameter set to "1"

Figure 110: Types of SPC charts

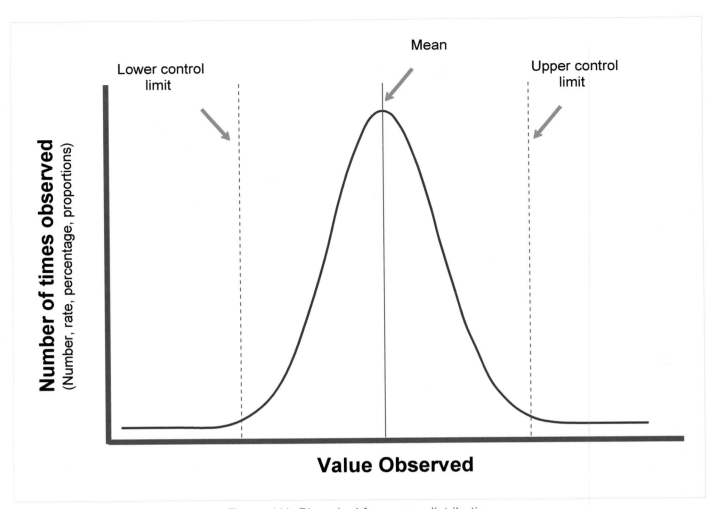

Figure 111: Binominal frequency distribution

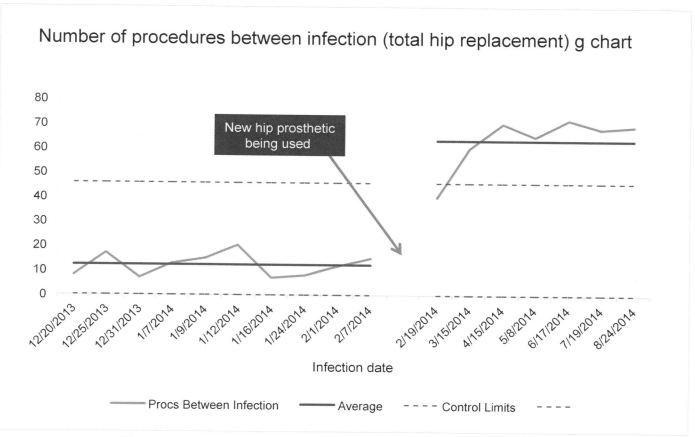

Figure 113: g chart example — number of procedures between infections

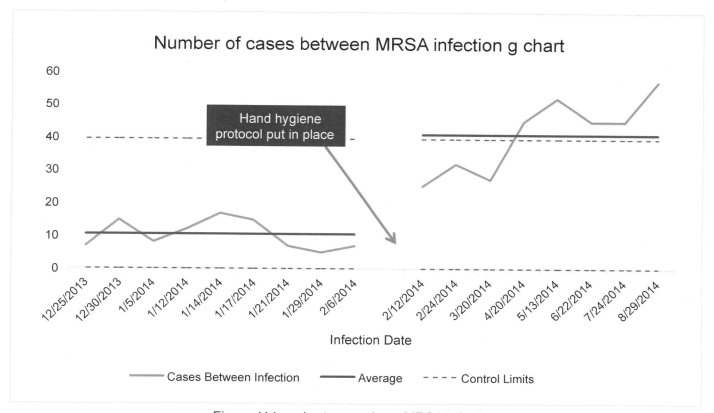

Figure 114: g chart example — MRSA infection

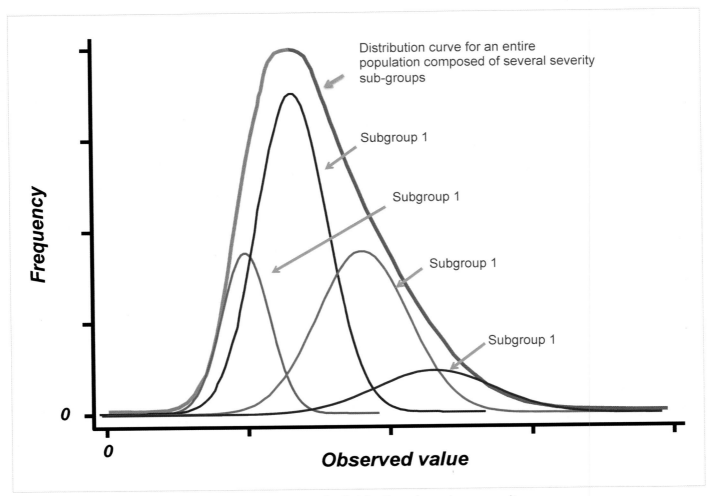

Figure 117: Parametric distributions based on severity

Empiric frequency distribution bar chart
(How the process behaves over many observations)

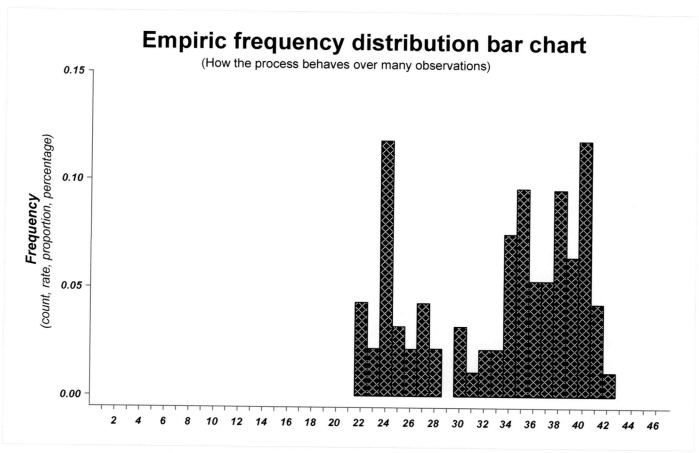

Figure 118: Shewhart's method for non-homogenous samples

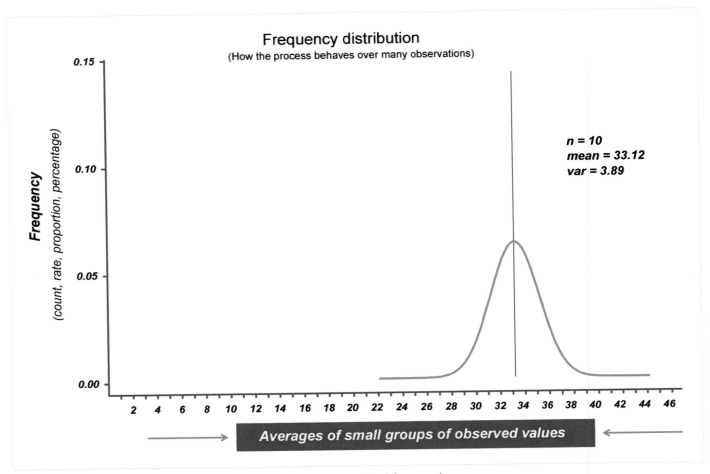

Figure 119: Shewhart's method for non-homogenous

Made in the USA
Las Vegas, NV
09 September 2022

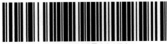